T0264033

Medicolegal and Ethical Issues in Neurology

Editors

JOSEPH S. KASS
MICHAEL A. RUBIN

NEUROLOGIC CLINICS

www.neurologic.theclinics.com

Consulting Editor
RANDOLPH W. EVANS

August 2023 • Volume 41 • Number 3

ELSEVIER

1600 John F. Kennedy Boulevard ● Suite 1800 ● Philadelphia, Pennsylvania, 19103-2899

http://www.theclinics.com

NEUROLOGIC CLINICS Volume 41, Number 3
August 2023 ISSN 0733-8619, ISBN-13: 978-0-443-18376-8

Editor: Stacy Eastman
Developmental Editor: Hannah Almira Lopez

© **2023 Elsevier Inc. All rights reserved.**

This periodical and the individual contributions contained in it are protected under copyright by Elsevier, and the following terms and conditions apply to their use:

Photocopying
Single photocopies of single articles may be made for personal use as allowed by national copyright laws. Permission of the Publisher and payment of a fee is required for all other photocopying, including multiple or systematic copying, copying for advertising or promotional purposes, resale, and all forms of document delivery. Special rates are available for educational institutions that wish to make photocopies for non-profit educational classroom use. For information on how to seek permission visit www.elsevier.com/permissions or call: (+44) 1865 843830 (UK)/(+1) 215 239 3804 (USA).

Derivative Works
Subscribers may reproduce tables of contents or prepare lists of articles including abstracts for internal circulation within their institutions. Permission of the Publisher is required for resale or distribution outside the institution. Permission of the Publisher is required for all other derivative works, including compilations and translations (please consult www.elsevier.com/permissions).

Electronic Storage or Usage
Permission of the Publisher is required to store or use electronically any material contained in this periodical, including any article or part of an article (please consult www.elsevier.com/permissions). Except as outlined above, no part of this publication may be reproduced, stored in a retrieval system or transmitted in any form or by any means, electronic, mechanical, photocopying, recording or otherwise, without prior written permission of the Publisher.

Notice
No responsibility is assumed by the Publisher for any injury and/or damage to persons or property as a matter of products liability, negligence or otherwise, or from any use or operation of any methods, products, instructions or ideas contained in the material herein. Because of rapid advances in the medical sciences, in particular, independent verification of diagnoses and drug dosages should be made.

Although all advertising material is expected to conform to ethical (medical) standards, inclusion in this publication does not constitute a guarantee or endorsement of the quality or value of such product or of the claims made of it by its manufacturer.

Neurologic Clinics (ISSN 0733-8619) is published quarterly by Elsevier Inc., 360 Park Avenue South, New York, NY 10010–1710. Months of issue are February, May, August, and November. Periodicals postage paid at New York, NY, and additional mailing offices. Subscription prices are $353.00 per year for US individuals, $809.00 per year for US institutions, $100.00 per year for US students, $433.00 per year for Canadian individuals, $980.00 per year for Canadian institutions, $489.00 per year for international individuals, $980.00 per year for international institutions, $210.00 for foreign students/residents, and $100.00 for Canadian students/residents. To receive student/resident rate, orders must be accompanied by name of affiliated institution, date of term, and the *signature* of program/residency coordinator on institution letterhead. Orders will be billed at individual rate until proof of status is received. Foreign air speed delivery is included in all *Clinics* subscription prices. All prices are subject to change without notice. **POSTMASTER:** Send address changes to *Neurologic Clinics*, Elsevier Health Sciences Division, Subscription Customer Service, 3251 Riverport Lane, Maryland Heights, MO 63043. **Customer Service: Telephone: 1-800-654-2452 (U.S. and Canada); 314-447-8871 (outside U.S. and Canada). Fax: 314-447-8029. E-mail: journalscustomerservice-usa@elsevier.com (for print support); journalsonlinesupport-usa@elsevier.com (for online support).**

Reprints. For copies of 100 or more of articles in this publication, please contact the Commercial Reprints Department, Elsevier Inc., 360 Park Avenue South, New York, New York, 10010-1710; Tel.: +1-212-633-3874; Fax: +1-212-633-3820, and E-mail: reprints@elsevier.com.

Neurologic Clinics is also published in Spanish by Nueva Editorial Interamericana S.A., Mexico City, Mexico.

Neurologic Clinics is covered in *Current Contents/Clinical Medicine, MEDLINE/PubMed (Index Medicus), EMBASE/Excerpta Medica, and PsycINFO, and ISI/BIOMED.*

Contributors

CONSULTING EDITOR

RANDOLPH W. EVANS, MD
Clinical Professor, Department of Neurology, Baylor College of Medicine, Houston, Texas, USA

EDITORS

JOSEPH S. KASS, MD, JD, FAAN
Professor, Department of Neurology, Menninger Department of Psychiatry and Behavioral Sciences, Center for Medical Ethics and Health Policy, Baylor College of Medicine, Houston, Texas, USA

MICHAEL A. RUBIN, MD, MA, FAAN
Associate Professor, Departments of Neurology and Neurological Surgery, Peter O'Donnell Jr Brain Institute, The University of Texas Southwestern Medical Center, Dallas, Texas, USA

AUTHORS

SASHA ALICK-LINDSTROM, MD, FAAN, FACNS, FAES
Departments of Neurology and Radiology, Peter O'Donnell Jr Brain Institute, The University of Texas Southwestern Medical Center, Dallas, Texas, USA

BERNA ARDA, MD, MedSpec, PhD
Professor and Head, Department of Medical Ethics, Faculty of Medicine, Ankara University, Turkey

ROY BERAN MBBS, MD, MHL
Conjoint Professor, University of New South Wales, Conjoint Professor, Western Sydney University, Sydney, Australia; Professor, School of Medicine, Griffith University, Queensland, Australia

DANIELLE FENG, MD
Department of Neurology, Harbor-UCLA Medical Center, Torrance, California, USA

ELIZABETH HEITMAN, PhD
Professor, Program in Ethics in Science and Medicine, Departments of Psychiatry and Applied Clinical Research, The University of Texas Southwestern Medical Center, Dallas, Texas, USA

JAMES C. JOHNSTON, MD, JD, FCLM (USA), FACLM (Aust), FAAN
GlobalNeurology®, Auckland, New Zealand; and San Antonio, Texas, USA; Department of Neurology, Addis Ababa University School of Medicine, Addis Ababa, Ethiopia

JOSEPH S. KASS, MD, JD, FAAN
Professor, Department of Neurology, Menninger Department of Psychiatry and Behavioral Sciences, Center for Medical Ethics and Health Policy, Baylor College of Medicine, Houston, Texas, USA

BRENT M. KIOUS, MD, PhD
Assistant Professor, Department of Psychiatry, Center for Bioethics and Health Humanities, University of Utah, Salt Lake City, Utah, USA

ABHAY KUMAR, MD
Associate Professor, Vivian L. Smith Department of Neurosurgery, McGovern Medical School at UTHealth Houston, Houston, Texas, USA

CHRISTOS LAZARIDIS, MD, EDIC
Departments of Neurology and Neurosurgery, MacLean Center for Clinical Medical Ethics, University of Chicago, Chicago, Illinois, USA

ARIANE LEWIS, MD
Departments of Neurology and Neurosurgery, NYU Langone Medical Center, New York, New York, USA

SUSAN P. RAINE, MD, JD, LLM, MEd
Professor of Obstetrics and Gynecology, Baylor College of Medicine, Houston, Texas, USA

JENNY RIECKE, MD
Assistant Instructor, Department of Neurology, Fellow, Department of Palliative Care, The University of Texas Southwestern Medical Center, Dallas, Texas, USA

RACHEL V. ROSE, JD, MBA
Principal, Rachel V. Rose – Attorney At Law PLLC, Affiliated Member, Center for Medical Ethics and Health Policy, Baylor College of Medicine, Houston, Texas, USA

MICHAEL A. RUBIN, MD, MA
Associate Professor, Departments of Neurology and Neurological Surgery, The University of Texas Southwestern Medical Center, Dallas, Texas, USA

THOMAS P. SARTWELLE, BBA, LLB
Hicks Davis Wynn, PC, Houston, Texas, USA

MEHILA ZEBENIGUS, MD
Department of Neurology, Addis Ababa University School of Medicine, Director, Yehuleshet Higher Clinic, Addis Ababa, Ethiopia

Contents

Informed consent (IC) is an ethical and legal requirement grounded in the principle of autonomy. Cognitive impairment may often interfere with decision-making capacity necessitating alternative models of ethically sound deliberation. In cases where the patient lacks decision-making capacity, one must determine the appropriate decision-maker and the criteria used in making a medical decision appropriate for the patient. In this article, I critically discuss the traditional approaches of IC, advance directives, substituted judgment, and best interests. A further suggestion is that thinking about sufficient *reasons* for or against a course of action is a conceptual enrichment in addition to the concepts of interests and well-being. Finally, I propose another model of collective consensus-seeking decision-making.

An increasing number of jurisdictions have legalized medical assistance in dying (MAID) with significant variation in the procedures and eligibility criteria used. In the United States, MAID is available for persons with terminal illnesses but is frequently sought by persons with neurologic conditions. Persons with conditions that cause cognitive impairment, such as Alzheimer dementia, are often ineligible for MAID, as their illness is not considered terminal in its early stages, whereas in later stages, they may have impaired decision-making capacity.

Medical futility is an ancient and yet consistent challenge in clinical medicine. The means of balancing conflicting priorities and stakeholders' preferences has changed as much as the science that powers the understanding and treatment of disease. The introduction of patient self-determination and choice in medical decision-making shifted the locus of power in the physician–patient relationship but did not obviate the physician's responsibilities to provide benefit and prevent harm. As we have refined the process in time, new paradigms, specialists, and tools have been developed to help navigate the ever-changing landscape.

Although the fundamental principle behind the Uniform Determination of Death Act (UDDA), the equivalence of death by circulatory-respiratory and neurologic criteria, is accepted throughout the United States and much of the world, some families object to brain death/death by neurologic criteria. Clinicians struggle to address these objections. Some objections have been brought to court, particularly in the United States, leading to inconsistent outcomes and discussion about potential modifications to the UDDA to minimize ethical and legal controversies related to the determination of brain death/death by neurologic criteria.

This article provides an overview of current malpractice trends in neurology as well as non-malpractice and forensic liability concerns. It is more important for clinicians to recognize the common patient care scenarios that are likely to precipitate lawsuits rather than memorize arcane legal principles. Therefore, this article offers an introduction to malpractice jurisprudence as well as a general overview of current litigation trends and a review of the role and duties of a neurologist serving as an expert witness. The next article highlights mitigation strategies for the most prevalent neurologic misadventures.

This chapter highlights the most frequently encountered neurological malpractice claims. The format is designed to provide a rudimentary understanding of how lawsuits arise and thereby focus discussion on adapting practice patterns to improve patient care and minimize liability risk.

Advances in electronic health record technology, the ever-expanding use of social media, and cybersecurity sabotage threaten patient privacy and render physicians and health care organizations liable for violating federal and state laws. Violating a patient's privacy is both an ethical and legal breach with potentially serious legal and reputational consequences. Even an unintentional Health Insurance Portability and Accountability Act of 1996 (HIPAA) violation can result in financial penalties and reputational harm. Staying complaint with HIPAA requires vigilance on the part of both individuals with legitimate access to protected health information (PHI) and the organizations handling that PHI.

Health care entities doing business with the federal government may run afoul of the False Claims Act and Anti-Kickback Statute not only when they directly submit fraudulent claims for government reimbursement but also when they create schemes that manipulate others into submitting (whether knowingly or unknowingly) illegal claims. In recent years, the Department of Justice is deploying these statutes to ensure that electronic health records are built and maintained with appropriate cybersecurity protections.

Women may acquire neurologic conditions during their reproductive years. As a result, the potential for pregnancy must be considered when selecting appropriate treatment of these women. Physicians who adhere to the standard of care through sound clinical judgment, use of shared decision-making, provide appropriate and timely consultation and follow-up, and clearly document all aspects of patient care minimize legal liability in the event of an unanticipated pregnancy resulting in fetal harm due to treatment with a teratogenic medication.

People living with neurologic conditions have historically been among the most marginalized groups in society. Advances in science and medicine have helped prevent, manage, or even cure many of these disorders. The byproduct of these successes is an aging population and members of the population at large with neurologic diseases and their sequelae. These sequelae may be imperceptible to others but often include a loss of skills or independence, which negatively impact a person's psychosocial and socioeconomic status, particularly when either activities of daily living are compromised or the affected individuals possess limited social and financial supports systems.

Global health programs engaging in isolated or short-term medical missions can and do cause harm, reinforce health care disparities, and impede medical care in the regions where it is so desperately needed. Related ethical, medical, and legal concerns are reviewed in this article. The authors recommend abandoning these ill-considered missions and focusing attention and resources on advancing neurology through ethically congruent, multisectoral, collaborative partnerships to establish sustainable, self-sufficient training programs within low- and middle-income countries.

NEUROLOGIC CLINICS

ISSUES OF RELATED INTEREST

Neurosurgery Clinics
https://www.neurosurgery.theclinics.com/
Neuroimaging Clinics
https://www.neuroimaging.theclinics.com/
Psychiatric Clinics
https://www.psych.theclinics.com/
Child and Adolescent Psychiatric Clinics
https://www.childpsych.theclinics.com/

THE CLINICS ARE AVAILABLE ONLINE!
Access your subscription at:
www.theclinics.com

Preface

Medicolegal and Ethical Issues in Neurology

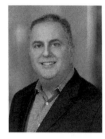   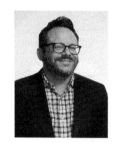

Joseph S. Kass, MD, JD   Michael A. Rubin, MD, MA
Editors

The fundamental principles guiding the legal and ethical practice of neurology continue to evolve and grow more complex. For this issue of *Neurologic Clinics*, we have assembled a group of national experts in both ethical and medicolegal issues who discuss a range of topics of interest to clinicians caring for individuals with neurologic conditions. We begin with a discussion of informed consent and decision making in patients who have lost decision-making capacity and therefore require specific attention when developing treatment plans. Medical assistance in dying is our next topic. While not permitted in all jurisdictions, medical assistance in dying has become relevant in the national conversation as even patients in states restricting such practices are able to access such pathways more easily in neighboring states. A comprehensive overview of medical futility and shared decision making from their ancient origins to contemporary medical practice comes next. The complex landscape of determination of death by neurologic criteria then receives specific coverage.

We then move away from ethical issues to review several core legal issues important to the clinicians caring for individuals with neurologic disease. We begin with a primer on medical malpractice and that includes a discussion of the duties and challenges of serving as an expert witness. With a strong theoretic background in place, the next article takes a deep dive into common scenarios that render neurologists vulnerable to malpractice claims and offers specific suggestions about how to improve patient care and avoid legal misadventure.

Having covered medical malpractice in depth, we then review other complex legal topics that render clinicians vulnerable to legal scrutiny: privacy and fraud. The article on privacy reviews HIPAA, explains relevant refinements to electronic privacy rules and medical record access requirements enshrined in the 21st Century Cures Act, and then discusses the implications of privacy laws and ethical conduct to clinicians' social

Neurol Clin 41 (2023) ix–x
https://doi.org/10.1016/j.ncl.2023.05.005
0733-8619/23/© 2023 Published by Elsevier Inc.

neurologic.theclinics.com

media use. Issues related to fraud are explored through a discussion of the False Claims Act and the Anti-Kickback Statute and includes a review of recent cases to provide clinicians with specific guidance about inappropriate behaviors.

This issue of *Neurologic Clinics* concludes with three articles addressing ethical and medicolegal issues germane to three particularly vulnerable categories of patients: individuals with neurologically based disability (whether visible or invisible), pregnant women and their fetuses, and individuals with neurologic disease in resource-poor countries.

Joseph S. Kass, MD, JD
Department of Neurology
Menninger Department of Psychiatry and Behavioral Sciences
Center for Medical Ethics and Health Policy
Baylor College of Medicine
7200 Cambridge Street
Houston, TX 77030, USA

Michael A. Rubin, MD, MA
Departments of Neurology and Neurological Surgery
Peter O'Donnell Jr Brain Institute
University of Texas Southwestern Medical Center
5323 Harry Hines Boulevard
Dallas, TX 75390-8855, USA

E-mail addresses:
kass@bcm.edu (J.S. Kass)
michael.rubin@utsouthwestern.edu (M.A. Rubin)

Informed Consent and Decision-Making for Patients with Acquired Cognitive Impairment

Christos Lazaridis, MD, EDIC[a,b,c,*]

KEYWORDS

- Informed consent • Capacity • Substituted judgment • Best interests
- Decision-making

KEY POINTS

- Informed consent (IC) is a cornerstone of contemporary medical ethics, grounded in respecting persons, their sovereignty, and autonomy.
- IC has three components: adequate informational content, voluntary decision-making, and capacity.
- Alternative models include decision-making based on advance directives, substituted judgment, best interests, and consensus seeking.

INTRODUCTION

Informed consent (IC), a core principle of modern medical ethics, is based on respect for persons and their autonomous decision-making. Philosopher John Stuart Mill formulated the moral grounding of IC when he stated, "Over himself, over his own body and mind, the individual is sovereign".[1] For bioethicists Beauchamp and Childress, "The autonomous individual acts freely in accordance with a self-chosen plan, analogous to the way an independent government manages its territories and establishes its policies".[2] It is this sovereignty over person and body that necessitates IC before performing any clinical activity affecting an individual. Whether a patient possesses or lacks decision-making capacity, the recommended framework for establishing goals of care is shared decision-making (SDM). The American College of

The author has no financial or other conflicts of interest in relation to this article. This article has not been published or submitted for review elsewhere.

[a] Department of Neurology, University of Chicago, IL, USA; [b] Department of Neurosurgery, University of Chicago, IL, USA; [c] MacLean Center for Clinical Medical Ethics, University of Chicago, IL
* Corresponding author. Division of Neurocritical Care, Department of Neurology, The University of Chicago Medicine, 5841 South Maryland Avenue, Chicago, IL 60637.
E-mail address: lazaridis@uchicagomedicine.org

Critical Care Medicine defines SDM as a collaborative process allowing either patients or their surrogates along with clinicians to make health care decisions together, taking into account both the best available scientific evidence and the patient's values, goals, and preferences.[3] This article analyzes different models of SDM for patients who lack capacity, specifically patients who lack decision-making capacity due to acute brain injury, disorders of consciousness (DOC), and advanced neurodegenerative conditions. I start by discussing IC, the gold standard model of interactions between patients and clinicians and the cornerstone of medical decision-making. The principle of autonomy, together with the related concept of sovereignty, underpins the requirement for IC. I then review alternative models of decision-making, all of which remain committed to the fundamental principle of respecting autonomy by developing treatment plans that the affected individual would endorse.

INFORMED CONSENT

IC has three critical and obligatory components. First, the informational content the health care professional or investigator provides must be adequate, and evaluated not only in terms of the breadth and accuracy of the data communicated but also in terms of the quality of the communication. Dense, technical content that neither patients nor surrogate decision-makers (SDMs) can understand fails to serve the intended function of having well-informed parties to the decision-making process. Second, the decision-maker must voluntarily engage with, accept, and endorse the plan of care. Although seemingly a straightforward condition, this component of the IC process may be compromised when decisions are time-sensitive and high stakes, as happens with acute brain injury. The pressure for a fast decision may undermine the quality of the exchange of information and the voluntary nature of decision-making. Finally, the decision-maker must have the capacity to receive, understand, and process the relevant information, weigh the risks and benefits of the recommended care plan, and consider the alternative courses of action with their attendant risks and benefits. Consent is considered fully informed when a capacitated patient to whom full disclosures have been made and who understands fully all that has been disclosed consents voluntarily to either treatment or participation on this basis.[4] Failure to establish IC, either directly or via surrogates, can be used to establish medical negligence as well as assault and battery.

This article focuses on decision-making *capacity* regarding context-specific decisions. Capacity determinations should not be based on one-time blanket assessments. Capacity may vary depending on the complexity and critical nature of the decision to be made. Patients who lack capacity to make highly complex decisions may still possess the capacity to make simpler ones. Capacity may vary over time, and an assessment at a certain time should not be assumed to carry forward. *Competency* is a global assessment and a legal determination to be made in court and will therefore not be addressed in this article. (N.B. Although ethicists commonly teach capacity as a physician's assessment and competency as a legal assessment, some statutes do refer to a patient's competency for medical decision-making as determined by a physician.)

What counts as adequate informational content? Three legal standards exist: the professional standard, the reasonable person standard, and the individual standard.[4] The *professional standard* calls for content that professionals or experts in a certain field would commonly consider as necessary or conventional to be disclosed, such as decisive data of a recent clinical trial that would strongly argue in favor of one course of action. Another example would be median life expectancy after a diagnosis or a therapeutic regimen. The *reasonable person standard* takes the patient's perspective and calls for informational content that a reasonable decision-maker would need to understand to come to a decision. The *individual standard* also takes the patient's perspective, but this time in a more personal and subjective manner where the specific values and preferences of an individual would have to be taken into account in shaping the informational content deemed pertinent for that individual.[5,6] All three standards, with their vague descriptions, have limitations, and their more concrete application for patients with either acute or chronic brain dysfunction can be challenging. Consider, for example, the case of a patient who presents with a large ischemic stroke, and the option of life-saving decompressive craniectomy (DC) needs to be discussed. What would these standards dictate regarding informational content? Would the professional standard be satisfied in discussing the literature on DC in addition to current guidelines? The issue with this suggestion is that the central question about the quality of survival is heavily nuanced and not directly answerable via an exposition of the clinical literature. Next, in terms of the reasonable standard, again is not clear how involved the conversation has to be to satisfy this criterion of reasonableness. Clinical trials and guidelines are relevant but should the clinical team's experience with prior patients also be disclosed? Finally, the individual standard would focus heavily on eliciting the patient's values and preferences—a requirement for all shared decision-making—as this decision must consider the patient's perspective on surviving but with a potentially significant neurologic disability. This standard requires that the informational content should be personalized to the extent possible. **Table 1** provides a summary exposition of the IC components, what they are, and the nuances involved.

ALTERNATIVES TO INFORMED CONSENT

If patient-derived IC is not feasible due to lack of decision-making capacity, what are the alternatives for ethically sound decision-making? IC is still required, but the issues here include who will be the most appropriate surrogate decision maker using the IC process to make decisions on behalf of the incapacitated patient and what criteria the surrogate should use in making an informed decision. The following models will be reviewed: Advance Directives; Substituted Judgment (SJ); Best Interests (BI) Standard; Parfit's Consent Principle (CP); and Consensus Seeking.

Advance Directives

One type of directive simply designates who the main surrogate is going to be if the need arises.[7] Living wills provide more guidance and instructions such as end-of-life preferences in terms of the extent and duration of mechanical support in the face of serious illness. Living wills are seldom available for younger patients with acute brain injury. A further problem is that even when a living will is available, often the guidance provided is generic, making its applicability and usefulness limited. This shortcoming becomes particularly evident as one considers the clinical nuances encountered among different acute brain injury pathologies and the great multidimensional uncertainty besides prognostic characterizing such clinical scenarios.[8] One of the great conundrums for decision-makers in these settings is the choice between preserving life versus promoting survival with a potentially unacceptable quality of life. Another interesting question, that has received attention in both the medical ethics and philosophical literature in relation to dementia, is the issue of precedent autonomy as established based on a choice memorialized in an advanced directive versus current interests of the patient with advancing dementia when these two conflict.[9–11] Another way to

Table 1
Components of informed consent, description, and nuances

Component	Description	Nuances
Informational Content	Legal standards • *Professional:* what is conventional among practitioners to disclose • *Reasonable:* what a reasonable person would consider pertinent • *Individualized:* what a particular person with a certain belief system and preferences would consider pertinent Benefits, risks, supportive arguments or data, and alternative courses of action ought to be provided	• Quality of communication is as important as content. Dense information in technical jargon does not serve the purpose • Unclear in practice how to satisfy the legal standards • Need to be aware of cognitive biases affecting all parties and the importance of acknowledging multidimensional uncertainty in decision-making after brain injury
Volition	• Consent must be free of external interference or undue influence • Decision as a manifestation of an individual's sovereignty and autonomy	• High-stakes time-sensitive decision-making may undermine the voluntary nature of decision-making or leave no choice • Cognitive biases and heuristics can be autonomy impairing
Capacity	• The ability to receive, understand, and process adequate information to weigh benefits, risks, consequences, and alternatives of a context-specific decision or course of action	• Often absent in patients with primary or secondary brain injury or disease • Should not be confused with competency which is based on a global assessment to be decided upon in court

express this conflict is between the autonomy of the earlier capacitated self and the well-being of the current incapacitated one. Arguments for either side have been articulated, with different authors giving more authority to autonomy and others to beneficence. Others have addressed the conflict via examination of personal identity as patients advance through stages of dementia. Here it is important to remember that individual decisions must be examined in terms of capacity, as the fact that a patient has been diagnosed with dementia does not immediately mean that they have lost all authority to make all decisions. Also, even if IC is not possible, one should attempt to establish capacity for either assent or dissent depending on circumstances.

Substituted Judgment

The surrogate's task is to reconstruct what the patient would have wanted under the circumstances at hand if the patient had decision-making capacity. One should pause here and consider the question about how easy it is to make decisions on behalf of someone else, even for a loved one or someone we believe we know well. Trivial choices with precedent may be easy to discern; nevertheless, the questions here are likely to be novel and concern life, death, disability, and even personal identity. Another extremely difficult hurdle to overcome is separating one's own belief systems, preferences, and reasons for action from those of the incapacitated patient. Separating personal beliefs from the beliefs of the incapacitated individual often becomes a difficult issue in the ICU, where SDMs may experience moral distress and fear decisional regret when withdrawing artificial support despite accepting that this course of action aligns with what the patients would have wanted.[12] SDMs must be informed that the underlying principle of SJ is respect for patient's autonomy rather than what SDMs personally think best under the circumstances. Being explicit that the surrogate is simply giving voice to the patient's decision can be very helpful in removing some of the emotional burden from SDMs.[13–15]

Besides theoretical and normative problems with SJ, empirical data questions SJ's ability to preserve patient's autonomy.[16] These data come from studies showing that a non-trivial percentage of people change their preferences over time and specifically about end-of-life care.[17] They also demonstrate a discordance between SDMs predictions and what patients actually want.[18] They also reveal that many patients prefer that decisions result from a combination of prior wishes and current input.[19,20] Torke and colleagues[16] proposed an alternative model of SJ based on the patient's life story and principle of respect for persons. In this modified type of SJ, surrogates would be asked not simply to predict the actual choices the patient would have made. Instead, SDMs are asked to make decisions that consider the individual's interests and values in the context of their current situation. In terms of principles, this modification deprioritize the principle of autonomy and focuses on the broader category of respect, which includes dignity and individuality, along with the duty to protect the incapacitated individual.

Best Interests

When employing the BI standard, the surrogate is being asked to consider what, all things considered, is the best course of action for the patient. The moral principle at work here is the principle of beneficence. What differentiates SJ from BI is that the latter is to be employed when precedent autonomy and prior preferences are unknown. As autonomy is not at play, beneficence takes over as the guiding principle. From a legal standpoint, "interests" refer to general goods such as the absence of or relief from pain and the recovery of somatic and mental health.[7] However, the conversation becomes nuanced if one thinks of interests in relation to theories of well-being.[21] For example, under a hedonistic account, a positive balance of either plea-sure or comfort over pain would provide positive well-being, and a course of action leading to such a state of affairs would be recommended. Recommendations could differ though if objective list theory guides decision-making, where regardless of what the outcome may bring in terms of comfort versus discomfort, the potential loss (or preservation) of an objective good, for example, the ability to acquire meaning-ful knowledge or to engage in rich interpersonal relationships, would determine the recommended plan of action.

Alternative ways of understanding BI have been proposed. Rebecca Dresser has suggested that instead of a generic conception of interests, we should look to commu-nity norms.[22] Robert Veatch has talked about "deep value" pairing, where SDMs, cli-nicians, and patients share a common value system as a guide to well-being and BI decision-making (in this article Veatch was making a larger argument to abandon IC).[23] Community norms could indeed be helpful in setting some boundaries on what kind of care is to be considered or recommended, yet such norms could still not entirely replace individualized decision-making. Such a move may be more apt for so-called unrepresented or unbefriended patients who lack either advanced direc-tives or SDMs.[24]

Parfit's Consent Principle

Derek Parfit's CP offers yet another paradigm for understanding both SJ and BI.[25] Parfit starts by examining Kant's claim that it is wrong to treat people in any way to which they cannot possibly consent. He offers several formulations of the CP such as "It is wrong to treat people in any way to which they could not rationally consent in the act-affecting sense, if these people knew the relevant facts, and we gave them the power to choose how we shall treat them". By act-affecting, Parfit means that people can either give or refuse consent if they have 'power over the proceed-ings,' because they will be treated in a particular way only if they consent. This formu-lation explains the moral significance—without direct reference to autonomy- of IC discussed earlier. A further formulation of the CP explains: "It is wrong to treat people in any way to which they would not have sufficient reasons to consent in the act-affecting sense" . This discourse about "sufficient reasons" is crucial for both SJ and BI deliberations. According to Parfit "when people know the relevant facts, they could rationally consent to some act just when these facts would give them suf-ficient reasons to consent. People have *sufficient* reasons to consent to some act when these reasons are not weaker than any reasons they might have to refuse con-sent".[25] The important new idea is that for both SJ and BI, an essential component of the deliberation should be about discovering reasons for and against different courses of action with the goal of finding a plan supported by *sufficient* reasons. An interesting difference between SJ and BI is that for SJ some of the reasons are "inter-nal" and subjective in the sense that they are generated by knowing the patient well and by taking their perspective—deploying information internally in relation to the pa-tient. BI recommendations are based on exclusively external, objective reasoning. For example, think of an individual who has been strongly committed to prohibiting with-drawal of life-sustaining measures. This attitude could serve as a strong or sufficient reason in determining how this person should be treated. Another example of an in-ternal reason leading to the opposite course of action would apply to someone whose life passion has been mountain climbing and is now faced with an injury that would preclude the individual from ever doing so again. Of course, one would have to weigh reasons for and against before determining that this reason would be sufficient in deciding to either withdraw or limit support. Parfit's CP conceptually enriches both

Table 2
Models of decision-making

Model	Ethical Principles	Applicability	Merits	Drawbacks
Informed Consent	Sovereignty, Autonomy, Respect	Capacity intact	Gold standard	Often impossible with cognitive impairment
Advance Directives	Sovereignty, Autonomy, Respect	Lacking capacity	Written representative instructions	Commonly does not exist. Hard to interpret in novel and nuanced scenarios after brain injury. Changing preferences over time (precedent autonomy vs. current interests)
Substituted Judgment	Sovereignty, Autonomy, Respect	Lacking capacity, having SDMs and known prior preferences	Autonomy preserving	Heavy burden for SDMs, variable quality of decision-making
Best Interests	Beneficence, Non-maleficence	Lacking capacity, having SDMs, unknown prior preferences	Focused on all things considered best course of action	Deliberations vary based on well-being theories and on what interests to prioritize
Consensus Seeking	Autonomy, Beneficence, Non-maleficence	Lacking capacity	Goal is to be more comprehensive. Support and coach SDMs. Protect patients.	Depending on the patient advocates could thwart autonomy. Untested in critical care.

Abbreviation: SDMs, surrogate decision-makers.

SJ and BI by adding considerations about the more general category of reasons, over the concepts of interests and well-being.

Consensus Seeking

The final decision-making model is *consensus seeking,* following the *mosaic approach* recently proposed by Joseph Fins.[26] Fins is motivated by thinking about patients with a DOC who may progressively be re-emerging as they regain degrees of their cognitive capacities. Fins is concerned with re-empowering the emerging patient. He is "seeking to achieve a proportionate and prudent balance between unbridled self-determination and conventional surrogate representation".[26] The reason why he calls it a *mosaic* is because there are several parties involved in the decision-making, including the emerging patient, the SDMs, the clinicians, and patient advocates. This collective is responsible for reaching a consensus that balances autonomy, non-maleficence, and the patient's BI. Both prior wishes and current preferences need to be included in the deliberations. Fins' model deserves special attention because it incorporates patient advocates into the discussion. Such advocate groups could conceivably be comprised of people representing disability groups, survivors of brain injury, and their caretakers, as well as independent health care professionals with relevant experience and expertise.[24,27] Potentially, hospitals or ethics committees could be tasked with creating such groups for prevalent conditions where SDM is known to be challenging—in acute brain and spinal cord injury and during critical illness—for example. This consensus-seeking, decision-making group aims to circumvent the problems identified above with AD, SJ, and BI models. Advocates can help SDMs in navigating novel and high-stress decision-making situations. Concern has been raised that family members may face extreme challenges in serving as patient advocates when they themselves are experiencing severe stress and are feeling under duress.[28,29] Also, advocates can potentially provide first-person lived experience data as well as empirical data in terms of decisional regret or the disability paradox.[30] Advocates can also mediate between clinicians and SDMs, finding the right balance in what information is presented and how it is communicated. Also, SDMs can describe patient's preferences, wishes, and life narratives to both clinicians and advocates; by having two groups with different (yet hopefully complementary) cognitive backgrounds attempting to reconstruct the best plan for the patient, a potentially more accurate and individualized set of recommendations can be proposed. This proposal is different from existing models that include advocates only for patients who are so-called unrepresented or unbefriended.[24] This consensus-seeking model has not been tested in critical care settings, and it certainly requires further analysis before implementation. Salient issues include the composition and training of the advocate group, the methodology of consensus, and safeguards against the advocate group thwarting SDMs' authority in representing the patient. **Table 2** provides a summary of all models discussed.

SUMMARY

Obtaining IC from a capacitated patient before clinical interactions is an ethical and legal requirement. The moral justification for this requirement is to respect persons, their sovereignty, and autonomy. Often, patients with brain injury or disease lack decision-making capacity. Different models of ethically sound decision-making are available and may apply depending on context-specific circumstances. To apply a model, one must decide who the parties involved in decision-making and what the decision-making criteria ought to be. This article has described and critiqued the conventional models of IC, advance directives, SJ, and the BI standard. A further suggestion is that thinking about *sufficient reasons* either for or against a particular course of action in addition to the concepts of interests and well-being enriches the discourse around what constitutes appropriate decision-making. Finally, another novel model of collective consensus-seeking decision-making includes patient advocates in the decision-making process and is patterned after Fins' mosaic approach and models recommended for unrepresented patients.

CLINICS CARE POINTS

- Decision-making capacity is context specific, and determinations should not be based on one-time blanket assessments as they may vary depending on how complex and critical the decision to be made is.

- Capacity may vary over time and an assessment at a certain time should not be assumed to carry forward.

- For patients with cognitive dysfunction and lack of capacity, we ought to engage in shared decision making with surrogates. This is a collaborative process that aims to incorporate best scientific evidence available with the patient's values, goals, and preferences.

- Future research should address the value of adding patient advocates into a consensus model of decision making.

REFERENCES

1. Mill JS. On liberty. In: Warnock M, editor. Utilitarianism/on liberty/essay on bentham. Glasgow: Fontana Press; 1990. p. 135, see also ch. 3.
2. Beauchamp TL, Childress JF. Principles of biomedical ethics. 6th edition. Oxford: Oxford University Press; 2008. p. 99–100.
3. Kon AA, Davidson JE, Morrison W, et al. Shared decision making in ICUs: an american college of critical care medicine and american thoracic society policy statement. Crit Care Med 2016;44(1):188–201.
4. Eyal N., Informed Consent, In: Zalta E.N, editor., 2019, The Stanford Encyclopedia of Philosophy (Spring https://plato.stanford.edu/archives/spr2019/entries/informed-consent/.
5. Berg JW, Appelbaum PS, Lidz CW, et al. Informed consent: legal theory and clinical practice. 2nd edition. New York: Oxford University Press; 2001. p. 46–52.
6. Beauchamp TL, Childress JF. Principles of biomedical ethics. 6th edition. Oxford: Oxford University Press; 2008. p. 122f.
7. Jaworska A. Advance Directives and Substitute Decision-Making. In: Zalta E.N. editor. The Stanford Encyclopedia of Philosophy (Summer; 2017. https://plato.stanford.edu/archives/sum2017/entries/advance-directives/.
8. Lazaridis C. Withdrawal of life-sustaining treatments in perceived devastating brain injury: the key role of uncertainty. Neurocritical Care 2019;30(1):33–41.
9. Dresser R. Life, death, and incompetent patients: conceptual infirmities and hidden values in the law. Ariz Law Rev 1986;28(3):373–405.
10. Dworkin R. Life's dominion: an argument about abortion, euthanasia, and individual freedom. New York: Knopf; 1993.
11. Jaworska A. Respecting the margins of agency: alzheimer's patients and the capacity to value. Philos Publ Aff 1999;28(2):105–38.

12. Andersen SK, Butler RA, Chang CH, et al. Prevalence of long-term decision regret and associated risk factors in a large cohort of ICU surrogate decision makers. Crit Care 2023;27(1):61.

13. Azoulay E, Pochard F, Kentish-Barnes N, et al. Risk of post-traumatic stress symptoms in family members of intensive care unit patients. Am J Respir Crit Care Med 2005;171(9):987–94.

14. Kentish-Barnes N, Lemiale V, Chaize M, et al. Assessing burden in families of critical care patients. Crit Care Med 2009 Oct;37(10 Suppl):S448–56.

15. Wendlandt B, Olm-Shipman C, Ceppe A, et al. Surrogates of patients with severe acute brain injury experience persistent anxiety and depression over the 6 months after ICU admission. J Pain Symptom Manag 2022;63(6):e633–9.

16. Torke AM, Alexander GC, Lantos J. Substituted judgment: the limitations of autonomy in surrogate decision making. J Gen Intern Med 2008;23(9):1514–7.

17. Auriemma CL, Nguyen CA, Bronheim R, et al. Stability of end-of-life preferences: a systematic review of the evidence. JAMA Intern Med 2014;174(7):1085–92.

18. Shalowitz DI, Garrett-Mayer E, Wendler D. The accuracy of surrogate decision makers: a systematic review. Arch Intern Med 2006;166(5):493–7.

19. Levinson W, Kao A, Kuby A, et al. Not all patients want to participate in decision making. A national study of public preferences. J Gen Intern Med 2005;20(6):531–5.

20. Kim SH, Kjervik D. Deferred decision making: patients' reliance on family and physicians for CPR decisions in critical care. Nurs Ethics 2005;12(5):493–506.

21. Crisp R. Well-Being", The Stanford Encyclopedia of Philosophy (Winter 2021 Edition), Zalta E.N. https://plato.stanford.edu/archives/win2021/entries/well-being/.

22. Dresser R. Precommitment: a misguided strategy for securing death with dignity. Tex Law Rev 2003;81(7):1823–47.

23. Veatch RM. Abandoning informed consent. Hastings Cent Rep 1995;25(2):5–12.

24. Pope TM, Bennett J, Carson SS, et al. Making medical treatment decisions for unrepresented patients in the ICU. An official american thoracic society/american geriatrics society policy statement. Am J Respir Crit Care Med 2020;201(10):1182–92.

25. Parfit D. On what matters: volume one (Oxford, 2011; online edn, Oxford Academic, 27 May 2015), chapter 8, Avaialble at: https://global.oup.com/academic/product/on-what-matters-9780199572809?cc=us&lang=en&. Accessed February 16, 2023.

26. Fins JJ. Mosaic decision making and severe brain injury: adding another piece to the argument. Camb Q Healthc Ethics 2019;28(4):737–43.

27. Chatfield DA, Lee S, Cowley J, et al. Is there a broader role for independent mental capacity advocates in critical care? An exploratory study. Nurs Crit Care 2018;23(2):82–7.

28. Kitzinger J, Kitzinger C. The 'window of opportunity' for death after severe brain injury: family experiences. Sociol Health Illness 2013;35(7):1095–112.

29. Kitzinger C, Kitzinger J. Grief, anger and despair in relatives of severely brain injured patients: responding without pathologising. Clin Rehabil 2014;28(7):627–31.

30. Ubel PA, Loewenstein G, Schwarz N, et al. Misimagining the unimaginable: the disability paradox and health care decision making. Health Psychol 2005;24(4S):S57–62.

Medical Assistance in Dying in Neurology

Brent M. Kious, MD, PhD

KEYWORDS

- Medical assistance in dying • Euthanasia • Amyotrophic lateral sclerosis
- Depression • Ethics

KEY POINTS

- An increasing number of states in the United States have legalized medical assistance in dying for persons with terminal illness.
- Persons with severe terminal neurologic conditions are especially likely to use medical assistance in dying if it is available.
- Complicated ethical issues can arise in providing medical assistance in dying to persons with terminal neurologic conditions because of deficits in cognition and motor function.

INTRODUCTION

Medical assistance in dying (MAID) is the process through which a physician or other health care professional[1] uses medical means—typically, a lethal dose of a medication or combination of medications—to intentionally produce the death of a patient at that patient's request.[2] MAID includes both physician-assisted suicide (PAS) and voluntary euthanasia.[3] In PAS, the medical provider writes a prescription for a lethal medication or combination of medications, which the patient ingests herself. In euthanasia, the medical provider directly administers the lethal medication following the patient's request.

The increasing global availability of aid in dying raises pressing ethical and clinical concerns for most physicians and other medical professionals, but serious and life-threatening neurologic conditions reaise unique issues because of their particular symptoms, including declining motor function, cognitive impairment, and the frequent presence of psychiatric comorbidity. Understanding the legal and ethical terrain associated with MAID in the United States is essential for practicing neurologists, palliative care physicians, and others caring for persons with chronic, debilitating, and terminal neurologic illness. This article reviews the US legal terrain surrounding MAID,

Department of Psychiatry, Center for Bioethics and Health Humanities, University of Utah, 501 Chipeta Way, Salt Lake City, UT 84108, USA
E-mail address: brent.kious@hsc.utah.edu

Neurol Clin 41 (2023) 443–454
https://doi.org/10.1016/j.ncl.2023.03.002
0733-8619/23/© 2023 Elsevier Inc. All rights reserved.

describing the typical approach to MAID in the United States, and then discusses alternatives to MAID, addressing specific issues related to several neurologic conditions and examining the impact of psychiatric illness on access to MAID.

DISCUSSION
Legalization of Medical Assistance in Dying

MAID has been legalized in the United States on a state-by-state basis. In 1994, Oregon passed the Death with Dignity Act (DWDA) by a ballot initiative, and despite efforts to overturn the act, it was implemented in 1997.[4,5] Subsequently, as of January 2023, a total of 10 US States plus the District of Columbia have legalized MAID.[6] **Table 1** lists the US jurisdictions where MAID has been legalized, the year legalization occurred, and the year that the law was enacted. Of note, MAID was legalized in Montana due to a decision of the state's Supreme Court rather than through legislation.[7] The status of MAID in Montana is contentious, with a bill recently proposed that would criminalize the practice.[8]

Many other countries have legalized MAID.[9] It is permitted in several European countries, such as Switzerland,[10] Belgium,[11] the Netherlands,[12] and Luxembourg.[13] It has also been legalized in stages in Canada.[14] **Table 2** lists jurisdictions outside of the United States where MAID has been legalized. The Benelux countries have legalized MAID through legislation, whereas in Switzerland, assisting in another person's suicide is not criminalized if it is not done from a selfish motive.[15] Accordingly, private right-to-die organizations, such as Dignitas,[16] Pegasos,[17] and Exit,[18] have arisen in Switzerland to provide end-of-life interventions.[19] The practice of MAID in Switzerland is especially relevant to US physicians as some Swiss right-to-die organizations permit non-Swiss citizens to receive their services; a number of US residents, some with a great deal of publicity,[20–22] have traveled to Switzerland for that reason, often under controversial circumstances.[23]

Multiple important differences exist between MAID in the United States and in Europe and Canada.[24] In the United States, MAID is restricted to persons with a terminal illness, which is generally taken to mean that death due to the illness is expected to occur within 6 months.[25] The US jurisdictions make no reference to whether the patient is *suffering* as a result of the illness.[26–34] In contrast, in some other jurisdictions,

Table 1
US jurisdictions that have legalized medical assistance in dying

State	Year MAID Legalized	Year MAID Available
Oregon	1994	1997
Washington	2008	2009
Montana	2009[a]	Not applicable
Vermont	2013	2013
California	2015	2016
Colorado	2016	2016
District of Columbia	2016	2017
New Jersey	2019	2019
Maine	2019	2019
Hawaii	2018	2019
New Mexico	2021	2021

[a] MAID is not legalized in Montana by statute but by a decision of the state's Supreme Court.

Table 2
Non-US jurisdictions that have legalized medical assistance in dying

Jurisdiction	Year MAID Legalized	Year MAID Available
Victoria, Australia	2017	2019
Western Australia, Australia	2019	2021
Tasmania, Australia	2021	2022
South Australia, Australia	2021	2023
Queensland, Australia	2021	2023
New South Wales, Australia	2022	2023
Austria	2022	2022
Belgium	2002	2002
Canada	2016	2016
Columbia	1997	1997
Germany	2020	2020
Italy	2019[a]	2022
Luxembourg	2008	2009
Netherlands	2001	2002
New Zealand	2020	2021
Spain	2021	2021
Switzerland	1942[b]	1942[b]

[a] Assisting suicide is permitted secondary to Constitutional Court ruling.
[b] Assisting suicide is not prohibited under the Swiss Penal Code.

MAID may also involve persons who have severe, unbearable, and irremediable suffering due to an illness, even if that illness is not terminal. In those jurisdictions, it is permissible to provide MAID to persons who are suffering severely as a result of chronic pain syndromes, severe but nonterminal neurologic conditions, or even mental illness.[35]

Another important international difference is that in many jurisdictions outside the United States, MAID can involve either PAS or voluntary euthanasia. In practice, however, euthanasia is more commonly recommended, perhaps because it is perceived as being easier for the patient.[36] In the United States, only PAS is currently permitted where MAID is legal.

The Practice of Medical Assistance in Dying in the United States

MAID laws in the United States are generally patterned after Oregon's DWDA,[26] although there are slight differences from state to state. Criteria for MAID and assessment procedures in Oregon are presented in **Box 1**.

In 2022, the Oregon Supreme Court upheld a suit from Dr Nicholas Gideonse, a family practice physician, arguing that the original law violated the rights of his patients who lived outside of Oregon.[37] Subsequently, Oregon has revised the DWDA to include nonresidents. This more inclusive approach may create complex legal dilemmas for Oregon physicians who provide MAID for patients who reside in states that do not permit MAID.

The DWDA indemnifies participating physicians and pharmacists from legal liability related to deaths occurring under the Act, provided they make a good faith effort to adhere to the Act's requirements. The Act forecloses disputes related to wills, contracts, or insurance, and stipulates that the patient's cause of death be reported as

---

Box 1
Criteria for medical assistance in dying and assessment procedures in Oregon

To be eligible for medical assistance in dying in Oregon, a patient must:
- Be 18 years of age or older
- Be a resident of Oregon[a]
- Be capable (able to make and communicate health care decisions)
- Have a terminal illness (death is expected within 6 months)

For MAID to be provided to an eligible patient, the following steps must occur:
- The patient must make two oral requests to the physician at least 15 days apart (in 2020, this was changed to permit patients whose life expectancy is < 15 days to make a second oral request less than 15 days after the first).
- The patient must submit a written request for MAID to the physician, signed by two witnesses (this may also be waived for persons whose life expectancy is < 15 days).
- A consulting physician must be appointed, both the prescribing physician and the consulting physician *must* confirm the patient's diagnosis and prognosis especially that the illness is terminal.
- Both the prescribing physician and the consulting physician *must* verify that the patient has decision-making capacity.
- If either physician believes that patient's judgment is impaired by "a psychological disorder or depression causing impaired judgment" the patient *must* be referred for evaluation and counseling by a psychiatrist or psychologist; the prescription may not be issued until the psychiatrist or psychologist determines, after counseling, that the patient is no longer suffering from impaired judgment due to the disorder.
- The prescribing physician *must* inform the patient of risks of the proposed intervention and of alternatives, for example, hospice.
- The prescribing physician *must* ask the patient to notify next-of-kin.
- The prescribing physician *must* ask the patient at the time of the second request if they wish to rescind their request.

[a]The residency requirement in Oregon was rescinded in 2022.

---

their underlying terminal illness rather than "suicide." The DWDA permits physicians to opt out of participation.

Deaths occurring under the DWDA have increased gradually. Since 1997, a total of 3,280 people in Oregon received MAID prescriptions, and 2,159 (66%) died of ingesting the medications. In 2021, MAID accounted for an estimated 0.59% of all deaths in Oregon.[38]

The clinical practice of MAID in Oregon and other states that permit it has evolved gradually. Although US MAID statues require an assessment of the patient's decision-making capacity, they do not lay out specific criteria for capacity assessment, instead treating capacity assessment as a matter of clinical judgment. Physicians and ethicists have accordingly espoused guidelines for assessing capacity before MAID.[39,40] The limited evidence available suggests that capacity assessment is typically informal,[41,42] but physicians who wish to formally assess capacity before MAID could use any of several instruments, such as the MacArthur Competence Assessment Tool.[43]

Most physicians who participate in MAID avoid proactively recommending it to their patients, instead relying on the patient to bring up the possibility.[44] Although this approach may be intended to avoid subjecting the patient to coercion or undue influence, it marks a significant departure from other domains of medical practice, where, typically, any plan of treatment must be discussed in comparison to alternatives.

A variety of medication regimens have been used for MAID, with changes sometimes being made because of the limited availability of preferred drugs. Physician readers who wish to learn more about prescribing for PAS, where it is legal, should consult their respective state departments of health for information about available training programs.

Reasons for seeking MAID vary widely, but in the United States, most patients report concerns related to the loss of autonomy and independence, rather than concerns about either pain or difficult physical symptoms.[38,45] These types of concerns contrast with the experience in many non-US jurisdictions, where relief of pain or other sources of suffering is more frequently cited as a reason for pursuing MAID.[46,47] These differences may reflect either variation in the clinical populations who request MAID or differences in how patients justify their request given different eligibility criteria.

Alternatives to Medical Assistance in Dying

MAID advocates sometimes regard the practice as part of a suite of end-of-life interventions[48] to be offered in addition to traditional palliative care and hospice.[49,50] They note that these different practices have shared goals.[51] Still, the relationship of MAID to other end-of-life interventions is controversial. The American Academy of Hospice and Palliative Medicine takes a position of "studied neutrality on MAID,[52] whereas the National Hospice and Palliative Care Organization supports individuals' right to choose MAID if legal.[53] The International Association for Hospice and Palliative Care supports the legalization of MAID only on the condition that a country already provides universal access to palliative care.[54]

Palliative care physicians and ethicists have argued that MAID is unnecessary if good palliative care is provided.[55,56] Historically, only a minority of palliative care providers have either supported MAID or been willing to participate,[57,58] although as MAID becomes more widespread this attitude may change.[59] Some evidence suggests that MAID recipients underutilize palliative care, although whether this is due to a lack of access or a lack of interest is unclear.[47]

Controversy also surrounds the relationship between MAID and other end-of-life practices, such as palliative sedation and voluntarily stopping eating and drinking (VSED). In palliative sedation, medical providers use sedating medications, including anesthetics, to lower a patient's consciousness to a "twilight state," thereby reducing their unpleasant symptoms; in some cases, sedation is continued to the point that the patient expires, either because of either suppression of cardiorespiratory function or dehydration due to the cessation of oral fluid intake.[60] Critics of palliative sedation—along with advocates for MAID—have argued that it is not morally distinct from MAID.[61] Advocates for palliative sedation who reject MAID note a morally salient difference between intentionally promoting death and merely causing death as a foreseen but unintended consequence of alleviating suffering.[62] Similar controversies apply to withdrawing life-sustaining or life-prolonging interventions for persons who are terminally ill; opponents of MAID often still support the withdrawal of life-sustaining treatments, noting that there is an important ethical difference between withdrawing a treatment and allowing natural death and actively engaging in a medical intervention (such as MAID) that causes death.[63,64]

VSED is seen as an alternative to MAID for patients who wish to hasten their own death but who either oppose MAID or who cannot access it. In VSED, the patient, often after the completion of an appropriate advance directive or living will, ceases to eat and drink.[3] VSED typically produces death within about 7 days.[65] Although some have observed that VSED seems less difficult to tolerate than expected,[66] patients may prefer MAID because of its rapidity, thereby avoiding discomfort associated with VSED, or because they fear that, facing profound hunger or thirst, they will change their minds.[67]

Special Issues for Persons with Neurologic Conditions

Several special issues arise for persons who request MAID because of terminal neurologic conditions as well as for persons for whom a non-neurologic terminal illness (eg, cancer) forms the basis of their request but who are simultaneously living with a serious neurologic condition. These issues vary by diagnosis, prognosis, and the types of disability associated with the diagnosis. Of note for neurologists, in February 2018, the American Academy of Neurology retired its position statement opposing MAID, leaving the decision "to the conscientious judgment of its members acting on behalf of their patients."[68]

Where MAID is legal, a minority of requesting patients have a terminal neurologic illness. In Oregon in 2021, 14.7% of recipients had a neurologic illness; the majority (9.2% of the total) had amyotrophic lateral sclerosis (ALS).[38] In Washington, 8.2% of MAID recipients had a neurodegenerative condition.[69] These figures suggest that ALS is significantly overrepresented among MAID recipients. If the prevalence of ALS is ~5 persons per 100,000 in the United States,[70] and the prevalence of terminal cancer is ~160 per 100,000,[71] and ~60% of MAID recipients have terminal cancer, then ALS is overrepresented by a factor of ~4.8. This overrepresentation may be because persons with ALS are especially afraid that they will lose independence or burden family members—a common concern for MAID recipients irrespective of diagnosis.[72,73]

Although MAID is often used by persons with ALS, the US approach, which permits only PAS, may be suboptimal for many individuals living with ALS. Individuals with ALS may be unable to ingest the pills necessary to complete the act either because of swallowing difficulties or difficulty handling the pills.[74] These difficulties are less likely in jurisdictions permitting euthanasia.[75]

Individuals diagnosed with Huntington disease (HD) may be interested in and may sometimes request MAID,[76,77] but they face difficulty with respect to timing; the average life expectancy after HD symptom onset may be as long as 15 to 20 years.[78] If a person recently diagnosed with HD wished to pursue MAID, she would be required under US laws to wait until her life expectancy was no more than 6 months. By the time her condition was "terminal", however, she would be more likely to experience severe psychiatric and cognitive symptoms,[79] including suicidal behavior,[80] which could then undermine her capacity to choose MAID. This dilemma has led some to explore the use of advance directives for euthanasia for HD patients in countries where euthanasia is permitted.[81] Similar issues arise with respect to other neurodegenerative conditions with psychiatric and cognitive symptoms, such as Alzheimer dementia, frontotemporal dementia, and Parkinson disease. Although there is increased use of advance directives for euthanasia in persons with Alzheimer dementia and related illnesses in some countries,[82] (eg, in Switzerland persons with early dementia have received MAID[22]) these practices remains controversial.[83–85]

Comorbid Mental Health Problems

Many individuals with terminal and severely life-limiting neurologic conditions, especially neurodegenerative conditions such as HD, have significant psychiatric symptoms. Conversely, some persons with preexisting psychiatric conditions develop terminal neurologic conditions. The conjunction of neurologic conditions and psychiatric symptoms has multiple ethical implications for MAID.

Comorbid psychiatric conditions may make MAID inaccessible to a patient with a terminal illness because the mental health disorder may undermine the individual's decision-making capacity. Patients with psychotic disorders such as schizophrenia may be especially likely to face this dilemma because an inadequately treated thought disorder reduces an individual's capacity to reason, understand, and appreciate information critical to informed medical decision-making. Even so, psychotic disorders do not invariably undermine decision-making capacity.[86] A person who has delusions in a single domain may still be able to make reasonable, well-informed decisions about whether to receive treatment for cancer. Thus, a patient's capacity should be assessed with respect to each specific decision.

Other psychiatric conditions—such as major depressive disorder, bipolar disorder, eating disorders, or personality disorders—may have less obvious effects on reasoning, though in many of these cases deficits in those aspects of decision-making capacity have been documented.[87,88] MAID laws in US jurisdictions reflect the view that depression itself, irrespective of its effects on reasoning, undermines decision-making capacity. Some have argued that depression reduces capacity by altering a people's values, so that they do not represent their "true self."[89,90] Depression, with its symptoms of hopelessness, increased isolation, and negative self-concept, may make MAID more appealing.[91] Most importantly, depression is associated with suicidal ideation, which could motivate MAID requests—though many have argued that there are significant differences between MAID and "ordinary" suicidal behavior.[92]

There is a growing controversy about the availability of MAID for persons with severe psychiatric illness. MAID has been available for persons suffering solely from psychiatric conditions in Belgium, Switzerland, the Netherlands,[93] and most recently Canada.[94] Some have even suggested that persons with severe, life-threatening anorexia nervosa should be eligible for MAID because they have a "terminal" psychiatric illness leading to death without treatment.[95]

SUMMARY

MAID is increasingly available in the United States and globally, although significant differences in approaches to the practice and eligibility criteria remain. Persons with severe and life-threatening neurologic conditions may have an increased interest in MAID and frequently use MAID where it is available. Enduring controversies about the general ethical permissibility of MAID, the relationship of MAID to palliative care and hospice, when physicians should promote alternative interventions, and the effect psychiatric and cognitive symptoms on access to MAID continue to inform societal discourse and legal responses to the practice.

CLINICS CARE POINTS

- Medical assistance in dying is currently legal in 10 states and the District of Columbia in the United States.
- Medical assistance in dying practice in the United States typically follows the model developed in Oregon, which legalized it in 1997.
- Persons with neurologic conditions such as amyotrophic lateral sclerosis are sometimes eligible for medical assistance in dying in the United States.
- Cognitive and psychiatric symptoms that impair decision-making capacity may complicate requests for medical assistance in dying from persons with severe and life-threatening neurologic conditions.

FUNDING

Greenwall Foundation Faculy Scholars Program.

DISCLOSURE

The author has no competing interests to declare.

REFERENCES

1. Pesut B, Thorne S, Stager ML, et al. Medical assistance in dying: a review of Canadian nursing regulatory documents. Pol Polit Nurs Pract 2019;20(3):113–30.
2. Emanuel EJ. Euthanasia. Historical, ethical, and empiric perspectives. Arch Intern Med 1994;154(17):1890–901.
3. Quill TE, Lo B, Brock DW. Palliative options of last resort: a comparison of voluntarily stopping eating and drinking, terminal sedation, physician-assisted suicide, and voluntary active euthanasia. JAMA 1997;278(23):2099–104.
4. Quill TE. The Oregon death with dignity act. N Engl J Med 1995;332(17):1174–5 [author reply: 1175].
5. Oregon Health Authority. Death with Dignity Act History. 2022. Available at: https://www.oregon.gov/oha/PH/PROVIDERPARTNERRESOURCES/EVALUATIONRESEARCH/DEATHWITHDIGNITYACT/Documents/history.pdf. Accessed January 31, 2023.
6. Compassion and Choices. In Your State. Available at: https://www.compassionandchoices.org/in-your-state. Accessed 06 June, 2022.
7. Bostrom BA. Baxter v. State of Montana. Issues Law Med 2010;26(1):7984.
8. Prohibit consent as a defense for physician-assisted suicide, SB 210, Montana Legislature, 68th Regular Session sess (Glimm C 2023). 2023. Available at: https://laws.leg.mt.gov/legprd/LAW0210W$BSIV.ActionQuery?P_BILL_NO1=210&P_BLTP_BILL_TYP_CD=SB&Z_ACTION=Find&P_SESS=20231. Accessed January 31, 2023.
9. Mroz S, Dierickx S, Deliens L, et al. Assisted dying around the world: a status quaestionis. Ann Palliat Med 2020;10(3):3540–53.
10. Guillod O, Schmidt A. Assisted suicide under Swiss law. Eur J Health Law 2005;12(1):25–38.
11. Deliens L, van der Wal G. Euthanasia law in Belgium and the Netherlands. Lancet 2003;362(9391):1239–40.
12. Weber W. Netherlands legalise euthanasia. Lancet 2001;357(9263):1189.
13. Watson R. Luxembourg is to allow euthanasia from 1 April. BMJ 2009;338:b1248.
14. Lemire F. Carter versus Canada: effects on us and our profession. Can Fam Physician 2015;61(8):728.
15. Hurst SA, Mauron A. Assisted suicide in Switzerland: clarifying liberties and claims. Bioethics 2017;31(3):199–208.
16. Dignitas. Dignitas. Available at: http://dignitas.ch. Accessed January 13, 2023.
17. Pegasos Swiss Association. Pegasos Swiss Association. Available at: http://pegasos-association.com. Accessed January 13, 2023.
18. Exit Deutsche-Schweiz. Who is Exit?. Available at: http://exit.ch. Accessed January 13, 2023.
19. Gauthier S, Mausbach J, Reisch T, et al. Suicide tourism: a pilot study on the Swiss phenomenon. J Med Ethics 2015;41(8). 611-607.
20. Prior R., My friend chose an assisted death in Switzerland. Her dying wish was to tell you why. CNN. 2020. Available at: https://www.cnn.com/2020/06/07/health/cindy-shepler-assisted-death-wellness-trnd/index.html. Accessed January 31, 2023.
21. Sperling N. A father chooses to end his life at 92. His daughter hit record. New York Times. 2022. Available at: https://www.nytimes.com/2022/10/06/movies/last-flight-home-documentary-ondi-timoner.html. Accessed January 31, 2023.

22. Bloom A, Love. A Memoir of Love and Loss. New York: Random House; 2022.
23. Hurley B. Arizona sisters who died by assisted suicide in Switzerland were 'tired of life'. The Independent. March 27, 2022. Available at: https://www.independent.co.uk/news/world/americas/arizona-sisters-assisted-suicide-switzerland-nitschke-b2045015.html. Accessed January 31, 2023.
24. Hanson RK, Mautz RD, Betts J, et al. Physician-assisted suicide and euthanasia: contrasting the American and European approaches. Journal of Leadership, Accountability and Ethics 2020;17(5):36–41.
25. Green K. Physician-assisted suicide and euthanasia: safeguarding against the "slippery slope"–The Netherlands versus the United States. Indiana Int Comp Law Rev 2003;13(2):639–81.
26. Death with Dignity Act, 127 (1994). Available at: https://www.oregon.gov/oha/ph/ProviderPartnerResources/EvaluationResearch/DeathwithDignityAct/Pages/ors.aspx. Accessed October 20, 2018.
27. Termination of Life on Request and Assisted Suicide Act, (2001). Available at: http://wetten.overheid.nl/BWBR0012410/2012-10-10. Accessed October 20, 2018.
28. Death with Dignity Act, 70.245 (2009). Available at: http://app.leg.wa.gov/rcw/default.aspx?cite=70.245. Accessed October 20, 2018.
29. Patient Choice at End of Life Act, Chapter 113 (2013). Available at: http://www.leg.state.vt.us/docs/2014/Acts/ACT039.pdf. Accessed October 20, 2018.
30. End of Life Act, AB-15 (2015). Available at: https://leginfo.legislature.ca.gov/faces/billTextClient.xhtml?bill_id=201520162AB15. Accessed January 31, 2023.
31. End-of-Life Options Act, 25-48 (2016). Available at: http://www.sos.state.co.us/pubs/elections/Initiatives/titleBoard/filings/2015-2016/145Final.pdf. Accessed October 20, 2018.
32. Death with Dignity Act, 21-577 (2016). Available at: https://www.deathwithdignity.org/wp-content/uploads/2015/11/DC-Death-with-Dignity-Act.pdf. Accessed October 20, 2018.
33. Our Care, Our Choice Act, HB 2739 (2018). Available at: https://www.capitol.hawaii.gov/session2018/bills/HB2739_HD1_.HTM. Accessed October 20, 2018.
34. Medical Aid in Dying for the Terminally Ill Act, P.L. 2019, c. 59 (2019). Available at: https://www.njconsumeraffairs.gov/Statutes/Medical-Aid-in-Dying-for-the-Terminally-Ill-Act.pdf. Accessed April 11, 2023.
35. Bolt EE, Snijdewind MC, Willems DL, et al. Can physicians conceive of performing euthanasia in case of psychiatric disease, dementia or being tired of living? J Med Ethics 2015;41(8):592–8.
36. Kouwenhoven PSC, van Thiel GJMW, Raijmakers NJH, et al. Euthanasia or physician-assisted suicide? A survey from the Netherlands. Eur J Gen Pract 2014;20(1):25–31.
37. Shivaram D. Physician-assisted death in Oregon is no longer limited to just state residents. Updated March 30, 2022. Available at: https://www.npr.org/2022/03/30/1089647368/oregon-physician-assisted-death-state-residents. Accessed January 23, 2023.
38. Oregon Health Authority. Oregon Death with Dignity Act 2021 Data Summary. 2022. Available at: https://www.oregon.gov/oha/PH/PROVIDERPARTNERRESOURCES/EVALUATIONRESEARCH/DEATHWITHDIGNITYACT/Documents/year24.pdf. Accessed January 31, 2023.
39. Werth JL, Benjamin GA, Farrenkopf T. Requests for physician-assisted death: guidelines for assessing mental capacity and impaired judgment. Psychol Publ Pol Law 2000;6(2):348–72.

40. Bourgeois JA, Mariano MT, Wilkins JM, et al. Physician-assisted death psychiatric assessment: a standardized protocol to conform to the California end of life option act. Psychosomatics 2018;59(5):441–51.

41. Preston R. Physician-assisted suicide-a clean bill of health? Br Med Bull 2017; 123(1):69–77.

42. Wiebe E, Kelly M, McMorrow T, et al. Assessment of capacity to give informed consent for medical assistance in dying: a qualitative study of clinicians' experience. CMAJ Open 2021;9(2):E358–63.

43. Grisso T, Appelbaum PS, Hill-Fotouhi C. The MacCAT-T: a clinical tool to assess patients' capacities to make treatment decisions. Psychiatr Serv 1997;48(11): 1415–9.

44. Buchbinder M. Aid-in-dying laws and the physician's duty to inform. J Med Ethics 2017;43(10):666–9.

45. Ganzini L, Goy ER, Dobscha SK. Oregonians' reasons for requesting physician aid in dying. Arch Intern Med 2009;169(5):489–92.

46. Wiebe E, Shaw J, Green S, et al. Reasons for requesting medical assistance in dying. Can Fam Physician 2018;64(9):674–9.

47. Munro C, Romanova A, Webber C, et al. Involvement of palliative care in patients requesting medical assistance in dying. Can Fam Physician 2020;66(11):833–42.

48. Wright AC, Shaw JC. The spectrum of end of life care: an argument for access to medical assistance in dying for vulnerable populations. Med Health Care Philos 2019;22(2):211–9.

49. Bernheim JL, Raus K. Euthanasia embedded in palliative care. Responses to essentialistic criticisms of the Belgian model of integral end-of-life care. J Med Ethics 2017;43(8):489.

50. Chambaere K, Bernheim JL. Does legal physician-assisted dying impede development of palliative care? The Belgian and Benelux experience. J Med Ethics 2015;41(8):657–60.

51. Hurst SA, Mauron A. The ethics of palliative care and euthanasia: exploring common values. Palliat Med 2006;20(2):107–12.

52. American Academy of Hospice and Palliative Care Medicine. Statement on Physician-Assisted Dying. Available at: https://aahpm.org/positions/pad. Accessed January 31, 2023.

53. National Hospice and Palliative Care Organization. Statement on Medical Aid in Dying. 2021. Available at: https://www.nhpco.org/wp-content/uploads/Medical_Aid_Dying_Position_Statement_July-2021.pdf. Accessed January 31, 2023.

54. De Lima L, Woodruff R, Pettus K, et al. International association for hospice and palliative care position statement: euthanasia and physician-assisted suicide. J Palliat Med 2016;20(1):8–14.

55. Gordijn B, Janssens R. The prevention of euthanasia through palliative care: new developments in the Netherlands. Patient Educ Couns 2000;41(1):35–46.

56. Rizzo RF. Physician-assisted suicide in the United States: the underlying factors in technology, health care and palliative medicine–Part one. Theor Med Bioeth 2000;21(3):277–89.

57. Marini MC, Neuenschwander H, Stiefel F. Attitudes toward euthanasia and physician assisted suicide: a survey among medical students, oncology clinicians, and palliative care specialists. Palliat Support Care 2006;4(3):251–5.

58. McCormack R, Clifford M, Conroy M. Attitudes of UK doctors towards euthanasia and physician-assisted suicide: a systematic literature review. Palliat Med 2012; 26(1):23–33.

59. Piili RP, Louhiala P, Vänskä J, et al. Ambivalence toward euthanasia and physician-assisted suicide has decreased among physicians in Finland. BMC Med Ethics 2022;23(1):71.

60. Quill TE. Myths and misconceptions about palliative sedation. Virtual Mentor 2006;8(9):577–81.

61. Juth N, Lindblad A, Lynöe N, et al. Moral differences in deep continuous palliative sedation and euthanasia. BMJ Support Palliat Care 2013;3(2):203–6.

62. Cohen-Almagor R, Ely EW. Euthanasia and palliative sedation in Belgium. BMJ Support Palliat Care 2018;8(3):307–13.

63. Harris J. Are withholding and withdrawing therapy always morally equivalent? A reply to Sulmasy and Sugarman. J Med Ethics 1994;20(4):223–4.

64. Sulmasy DP, Sugarman J. Are withholding and withdrawing therapy always morally equivalent? J Med Ethics 1994;20(4):218–22 [discussion: 223-4].

65. Bolt EE, Hagens M, Willems D, et al. Primary care patients hastening death by voluntarily stopping eating and drinking. Ann Fam Med 2015;13(5):421–8.

66. Wax JW, An AW, Kosier N, et al. Voluntary Stopping Eating and Drinking. J Am Geriatr Soc 2018;66(3):441–5.

67. Menzel PT. Merits, Demands, and Challenges of VSED. Narrat Inq Bioeth 2016; 6(2):121–6.

68. Russell JA, Epstein LG, Bonnie RJ, et al. Lawful physician-hastened death: AAN position statement. Neurology 2018;90:420–2.

69. Washington State Department of Health. 2021 Death with Dignity Act Report. 2022. Available at: https://doh.wa.gov/sites/default/files/2022-11/422-109-DeathWith DignityAct2021.pdf?uid=63d857ebd8e8c. Accessed January 31, 2023.

70. Mehta P, Kaye W, Raymond J, et al. Prevalence of amyotrophic lateral sclerosis - United States, 2015. MMWR Morb Mortal Wkly Rep 2018;67(46):1285–9.

71. National Cancer Institute. Cancer Statistics. 2020. Available at: https://www. cancer.gov/about-cancer/understanding/statistics#:~:text=The%20cancer%20 death%20rate%20(cancer,and%20135.7%20per%20100%2C000%20women. Accessed January 31, 2023.

72. Achille MA, Ogloff JR. Attitudes toward and desire for assisted suicide among persons with amyotrophic lateral sclerosis. Omega (Westport) 2003;48(1):1–21.

73. Ganzini L, Johnston WS, McFarland BH, et al. Attitudes of patients with amyotrophic lateral sclerosis and their care givers toward assisted suicide. N Engl J Med 1998;339(14):967–73.

74. Norris SP, Likanje M-FN, Andrews JA. Amyotrophic lateral sclerosis: Update on clinical management. Curr Opin Neurol 2020;33(5):641–8.

75. Maessen M, Veldink JH, Onwuteaka-Philipsen BD, et al. Euthanasia and physician-assisted suicide in amyotrophic lateral sclerosis: a prospective study. J Neurol 2014;261(10):1894–901.

76. Regan L, Preston NJ, Eccles FJR, et al. The views of adults with Huntington's disease on assisted dying: a qualitative exploration. Palliat Med 2018;32(4):708–15.

77. Booij SJ, Tibben A, Engberts DP, et al. Thinking about the end of life: a common issue for patients with Huntington's disease. J Neurol 2014;261(11):2184–91.

78. Solberg OK, Filkuková P, Frich JC, et al. Age at death and causes of death in patients with Huntington disease in Norway in 1986-2015. J Huntingtons Dis 2018; 7(1):77–86.

79. McAllister B, Gusella JF, Landwehrmeyer GB, et al. Timing and impact of psychiatric, cognitive, and motor abnormalities in Huntington disease. Neurology 2021; 96(19):e2395–406.

80. van Duijn E, Fernandes AR, Abreu D, et al. Incidence of completed suicide and suicide attempts in a global prospective study of Huntington's disease. BJPsych Open 2021;7(5):e158.

81. Booij SJ, Rödig V, Engberts DP, et al. Euthanasia and advance directives in Huntington's disease: qualitative analysis of interviews with patients. J Huntingtons Dis 2013;2(3):323–30.

82. Marijnissen RM, Chambaere K, Oude Voshaar RC. Euthanasia in dementia: a narrative review of legislation and practices in the Netherlands and Belgium. Front Psychiatr 2022;13:857131.

83. Mangino DR, Nicolini ME, De Vries RG, et al. Euthanasia and Assisted Suicide of Persons With Dementia in the Netherlands. Am J Geriatr Psychiatry 2020;28(4):466–77.

84. Cohen-Almagor R. First do no harm: euthanasia of patients with dementia in Belgium. J Med Philos 2016;41(1):74–89.

85. Battin MP, Kious BM. Ending one's life in advance. Hastings Cent Rep 2021;51(3):37–47.

86. Dunn LB. Capacity to consent to research in schizophrenia: the expanding evidence base. Behav Sci Law 2006;24(4):431–45.

87. Hindmarch T, Hotopf M, Owen GS. Depression and decision-making capacity for treatment or research: a systematic review. BMC Med Ethics 2013;14(1):54.

88. Owen GS, Martin W, Gergel T. Misevaluating the future: affective disorder and decision-making capacity for treatment - a temporal understanding. Psychopathology 2018;51(6):371–9.

89. Rudnick A. Depression and competence to refuse psychiatric treatment. J Med Ethics 2002;28(3):151–5.

90. Elliott C. Caring about risks: are severely depressed patients competent to consent to research? Arch Gen Psychiatry 1997;54(2):113–6.

91. Blikshavn T, Husum TL, Magelssen M. Four reasons why assisted dying should not be offered for depression. J Bioeth Inq 2017;14(1):151–7. https://doi.org/10.1007/s11673-016-9759-4.

92. Creighton C., Cerel J. and Battin M., Statement of the American Association of Suicidology:"Suicide" is not the same as "Physician aid in dying", *American Association of Suicidology*, 2017. Available from: https://ohiooptions.org/wp-content/uploads/2016/02/AAS-PAD-Statement-Approved-10.30.17-ed-10-30-17.pdf. Accessed April 11, 2023.

93. Kim SYH, De Vries RG, Peteet JR. Euthanasia and assisted suicide of patients with psychiatric disorders in the Netherlands 2011 to 2014. JAMA Psychiatr 2016;73(4):362–8.

94. Health Canada. Final Report of the Expert Panel on MAiD and Mental Illness. 2022. Available at: https://www.canada.ca/en/health-canada/corporate/about-health-canada/public-engagement/external-advisory-bodies/expert-panel-maid-mental-illness/final-report-expert-panel-maid-mental-illness.html. Accessed September 22, 2022.

95. Gaudiani JL, Bogetz A, Yager J. Terminal anorexia nervosa: three cases and proposed clinical characteristics. Journal of Eating Disorders 2022;10(1):1–14.

Futility and Shared Decision-Making

Michael A. Rubin, MD, MA[a,b,*], Jenny Riecke, MD[a,c],
Elizabeth Heitman, PhD[d,e]

KEYWORDS

- Futility • Clinical judgment • patient centered care • Shared decision-making

KEY POINTS

- Futility and the appropriateness of a medical treatment have been essential considerations since the ancient origins of healing as a profession.
- Attempts to philosophically or scientifically define a threshold that treatment should not be offered have been contentious.
- As medicine has turned to patient-centered care, so has the locus of decision-making authority shifted towards the patient's right of self-determination, however, clinicians still have a duty to advocate for what they believe is in the patient's best medical interest.
- The growth of palliative care medicine and decision-making tools has enhanced patient autonomy by helping them navigate through complex decisions.

ANCIENT ORIGINS OF THE CONCEPT OF MEDICAL FUTILITY

The dynamic tension between the fundamental precepts of doing good, *beneficence*, and not doing harm, *nonmaleficence*, has long characterized the ethics of medicine. Since its origins, Western medicine's ethical duties to patients have depended on the physician's *clinical judgment*—astute powers of observation, in-depth knowledge, and critical discernment—to diagnose and treat disease in the right way and at the right time. Historically, clinical judgment has included knowing when medicine offers no benefit and therefore when not to attempt to intervene in the course of illness, even in the face of death.

[a] Department of Neurology, University of Texas Southwestern Medical Center, 5323 Harry Hines Boulevard, Dallas, TX 75390-8855, USA; [b] Department of Neurological Surgery, University of Texas Southwestern Medical Center, 5323 Harry Hines Boulevard, Dallas, TX 75390-8855, USA; [c] Department of Palliative Care, University of Texas Southwestern Medical Center, 5323 Harry Hines Boulevard, Dallas, TX 75390-8855, USA; [d] Program in Ethics in Science and Medicine, Department of Psychiatry, University of Texas Southwestern Medical Center, 5323 Harry Hines Boulevard, NC5.832, Dallas, TX 75390-9070, USA; [e] Department of Applied Clinical Research, University of Texas Southwestern Medical Center, 5323 Harry Hines Boulevard, NC5.832, Dallas, TX 75390-9070, USA

* Corresponding author. Department of Neurology, University of Texas Southwestern Medical Center, 5323 Harry Hines Boulevard, Dallas, TX 75390-8855.
E-mail address: Michael.Rubin@UTSouthwestern.edu

Neurol Clin 41 (2023) 455–467
https://doi.org/10.1016/j.ncl.2023.03.005
0733-8619/23/© 2023 Elsevier Inc. All rights reserved.
neurologic.theclinics.com

Attention to the limits of medicine is a core theme in the Hippocratic Corpus.[1] The Hippocratic treatise commonly known as *The Art,* written between 430 and 330 BCE, defines the goal of medicine in terms of both its healing power and its absolute limits:

> *I will define what I conceive medicine to be. In general terms, it is to do away with the sufferings of the sick, to lessen the violence of their diseases, and to refuse to treat those who are overmastered by their diseases, realizing that in such cases medicine is powerless.*[2]

The Art's author defends physicians' refusal to take "desperate cases" with a denunciation of critics who insist that doctors should attempt cures when none is possible:

> *(I)f a man demand from an art a power that does not belong to the art, or from nature a power over what does not belong to nature, his ignorance is more aligned to madness than to lack of knowledge. Whenever, therefore, a man suffers from an ill which is too strong for the means at the disposal of medicine, he must surely not even expect that it can be overcome by medicine.*[2]

A large selection of the Hippocratic writings, particularly *Epidemics, Prognosis, and Regimens in Acute Diseases,* provide a detailed account of the various signs of illness and the indications for when and how to intervene.[1] Many of these texts also describe signs of when it is too late to do so. Hippocratic physicians recognized and admitted openly that it was "impossible to cure all patients" and that many of the cases they undertook ended in the patient's death.[1] The author of *Epidemics* advised fellow physicians that by "realizing and announcing beforehand which patients were going to die," the doctor "would absolve himself of any blame" for the death. More importantly, he noted that it was essential to pay "much attention to prognosis," to "know to what extent (diseases) exceed the strength of the body and have a thorough acquaintance with their future course."[1] By doing so, *Epidemics* advised, "one (might) become a good physician and justly win high fame."[1] In contrast, the Hippocratic writings lamented that medical charlatans promised cures to all diseases equally and that "laymen, far from recognizing those who excel in the treatment of acute diseases, generally praise or blame any cure that is different and give such quack their reputations as physicians."[1]

CONTEMPORARY CONCEPTUAL CHANGES

For some 2500 years, the physician's clinical judgment was the foundation for medical decision-making. Clinical judgment in medical care underwent a major transformation in the twentieth century with the increase of the scientific method in research, an improved understanding of disease etiology, and the development of an ever-growing array of new interventions and technologies that reversed once fatal conditions.[3,4] Clinical judgment became associated with the physician's subjectivity, bias, and error as modern research methodology emphasized the value of evidence-based medicine.[3] Almost simultaneously, the sustained development of new medical treatments—with and without a strong evidence base—made physicians increasingly reluctant to say that there was nothing they could do for patients with fatal conditions. By the 1970s, physicians were often unwilling to say that a patient was dying.[5,6]

In the second half of the twentieth century, US medicine in particular saw the effects of what economist Victor Fuchs called the *technological imperative,* the perceived need to use any available technology that offered the possibility of benefit, whether in medical diagnosis or treatment.[4,7] As physicians and the public assessed medicine's commitment to beneficence and nonmaleficence, many concluded that taking action was morally superior to inaction and that patients deserved every chance at life.[4] Seriously ill patients and their families increasingly sought specific medical interventions where none had been possible before, and physicians abandoned medicine's traditional acceptance of limits as they adopted a technological approach to illness and death.[5,7,8]

Nonetheless, by the late 1960s, some seriously ill patients struggled against physicians' efforts to postpone death, especially when physicians' attempts at rescue medicine left dying patients dependent on medical technology and unable to advocate for themselves. Over the next 4 decades, professional and public consideration of the ethical practice of medicine often focused on the goals and proper use of technology at the end of life as well as on who should decide the proper course of treatment in complex medical situations.[4,9] Questions about the limits of interventions that for centuries had been matters for the physician's clinical judgment and moral discretion became issues for debate and legal documentation by patients, regulatory oversight, and the courts.[9,10] The legal consensus that emerged was that physicians are not legally or ethically bound to provide futile treatment, but the ambiguity of what constitutes medical futility remains a problem.

DEFINITIONS OF FUTILITY: QUANTITATIVE AND QUALITATIVE MEASURES

In the clinical tension and social debate over the limits of medicine at the end of life, physicians and medical ethicists in the early 1990s attempted to integrate principles of evidence-based medicine and physicians' clinical experience to define standards for determining that a given intervention was "futile" in a particular context. Schneiderman and colleagues proposed a medical treatment that had been "useless" in the last 100 similar cases, and where theoretical successful outcome was not systematically reproducible, should be regarded as futile—an "action that cannot achieve the goals of the action, no matter how often repeated."[11] Under such circumstances, the treating doctor would have no duty to present the intervention to the patient or patient's surrogate decision-maker as an option and would not be obliged to provide that intervention in response to specific demands.

Through the 1990s, a series of others attempted to refine this definition and the relationship between the *quantitative* improbability of a desired outcome and the *qualitative* utility or benefit of that outcome in a given context.[11,12] Schneiderman later recommended combining quantitative and quantitative approaches to establish a workable, practical standard for specific cases, defining futility as "the unacceptably low likelihood of achieving an effect that the patient has the capacity to appreciate as a benefit."[13] Nonetheless, as Brody and Halevy argued, the challenge of defining futility was the need for *prospective* determination, before a potentially harmful and ineffective treatment might be tried. None of the proposed definitions, they noted, provided the clarity needed to allow physicians "to unilaterally limit life-prolonging interventions in certain cases while preserving the rights of patients and surrogates to decide about the provision of such interventions in other cases."[14]

Moving away from unilateral decision-making about futility, in the late 1990s, the American Medical Association (AMA) and multiple institutions proposed procedural approaches to evaluating potential futile or otherwise inappropriate treatment that could address patients' and families' values as well as medical evidence.[15] Over the next decade, debate continued over what futility means and how to operationalize a system to recognize and enforce limits. In 2014, a contemporary consensus guideline group was formed, involving experts from several medical professional societies, including the American Thoracic Society, American Association for Critical Care Nurses, American College of Chest Physicians, and the European Society for Intensive Care Medicine, and the Society of Critical Care Medicine. They recommended that medical institutions develop strategies to *prevent* decision conflicts and restrict the use of the word "futility" to its physiologic sense with other treatments categorized as "potentially inappropriate." Importantly, they emphasized the crucial role of the medical profession leading public engagement on when life-sustaining technologies should be limited.[16] Critics might argue that these guidelines diminish the importance of physicians' recommendations in decision-making, but they did definitively create a common starting point supported by a wide group of clinical stakeholders.

SOCIAL UPHEAVAL SHIFTS THE LOCUS OF POWER

The cultural changes of the middle to late twentieth century led to a shift in the locus of power in the physician–patient relationship. Physician-centered medical practice continued through the early part of this period. Innovations after WWII increased the effectiveness of medical treatment and elevated public trust in physicians as authority figures, which led to both physician-driven decision-making and physician control of information. With a public image of physicians as benevolent father figures, medical practice remained most consistent with the Hippocratic tradition that limited the patient's role to the recipient of care.[17,18]

The consumer rights movement, revelations of research atrocities, and rising costs of health care as well as a social shift toward questioning blind loyalty to authority shifted the power balance toward the patient. The National Commission for the Protection of Human Subjects of Biomedical and Behavioral Research's 1979 *Belmont Report* and Beauchamp and Childress's 1979 seminal work, "Principles of Biomedical Ethics" popularized the ethical principles relevant to Western ethical medical practice, emphasizing not only the beneficence and nonmaleficence of the Hippocratic age but also bringing attention to autonomy and justice.[19,20]

Although contemporary ethics committees may be more familiar with requests to address patient demands to continue treatments deemed potentially inappropriate, the influential legal cases of the age established the right of patients or their surrogates to refuse medical interventions. Although this source of conflict may sound odd in the twenty-first century, physicians and hospitals faced a real fear that either withdrawing or withholding life-sustaining treatment would be considered not only bad medicine but also criminal homicide. The increase of advance directives and passage of the Patient Self-Determination Act of 1991 informing patients of their right to establish their advance directives made the planned withdrawal of life support a norm, and respect for patients' role in decision-making a legal requirement for hospitals, nursing homes, home health agencies, and hospice centers.[9]

PATIENT-CENTERED MEDICAL CARE

This upheaval has since been labeled "patient-centered" medical care, emphasizing that the patient, rather than the clinician, is the locus of power in the patient–physician relationship. The Institute of Medicine has defined patient-centered care as, "patient involvement, individualization and education" and established patient-centeredness as a quality metric.[21] The Picker Foundation and Commonwealth Fund designated eight dimensions of Patient-Centered Care including:[22]

- Respect for patients' values, preferences, and expressed needs
- Coordination and integration of care
- Information, communication, and education
- Physical comfort
- Emotional support and alleviation of fear and anxiety

- Involvement of family and friends
- Transition and continuity
- Access to care

The shift toward patient-centered care does not obviate physicians' duty to advocate for medical treatments they judge to be in their patients' best medical interest. Rather, it invites the patient to be part of the discussion of what constitutes "best medical interest" and why. In addition, physicians may grow concerned that they can be compelled to act in ways that are inconsistent with either their professional judgment or their moral worldview. Recasting this concern as "professional autonomy," some critics of patient-centered care have attempted to establish that physicians have a right to self-determination equal to that of their patients.[23] Although physicians' moral integrity is essential to professional ethics, it is more traditionally understood as the right to remove oneself from a professional relationship in circumstances where either the patient's requests for treatment or overall behavior are not morally acceptable to the clinician. The framing of such professional conscience as professional autonomy does not support the physician imposing care plans against the will of the patient.

Although the scholarly literature substantiates the ethics and practical value of a patient-centered relationship, empirical evidence also supports the observation that not every patient wants the burden of medical decision-making or a patient-centered communication style. For example, a group of 250 participants who viewed videorecorded scenarios demonstrating both patient-centered communication and a more physician-directed, biomedically driven approach were split on which they preferred: 69% (95% CI 63 to 75) preferred the patient-centered style, but the large remainder preferred the physician-directed approach.[24]

Most recently, the shift to patient-centered care and has culminated in the "21st Century Cures Act" which requires immediate availability to patients of their medical information including objective data and their physicians' documentation. This new demand for transparency has led to some concern that patient's immediate access to information without interpretation of its context and meaning from a physician may confuse, frustrate, and frighten patients. Potentially most important for decision-making, it is possible that by the time the clinician presents treatment options, the patient may already be invested in a preference for care that is not justified by the facts of his or her illness.[25]

THE DEVELOPMENT OF SHARED MEDICAL DECISION-MAKING

The term *shared decision-making* anticipated patient-centered care by a few decades but is based on the same paradigm shift. First used in 1982 in the report "Ethical and Legal Implications of Informed Consent in the Patient-Practitioner Relationship" by the President's Commission for the Study of Ethical Problems in Medicine and Biomedical and Behavioral Research, the term "shared decision-making" was used to emphasize the importance of the clarifying values, sharing information, and implementing evidence-based care plans when treating serious illness and at the end of life.[22] The importance of shared decision-making in clinical neurosciences is recognized in many papers in neurocritical care, multiple sclerosis, epilepsy, and neurosurgery, among others.[22,26–28]

Many models of shared decision-making are available in the contemporary literature, including the "Collaborative Autonomy" model that emphasizes building a partnership to empower patient self-determination. In this model, the clinician's role is to assess the patient's understanding of the clinical scenario, elicit their values, discuss feasible options, after which the physician is encouraged to recommend a course of action most medically appropriate and most consistent with the patient's stated goals.

Depending on the nature and complexity of the decision, multiple iterations of the process may be needed to reach consensus on a plan of action.[29] The physician's responsibilities across the many different shared decision-making models have common elements: learning about the patient, describing treatment options, considering the patient's preferences, tailoring information to the relevant decision, deliberating, creating choice awareness, and making a decision.[30] Too often, physicians misinterpret the process of shared decision-making as an obligation to offer the full range of options without expressing a professional opinion and then yield completely to the patient. Such an approach would be a significant ethical lapse in that failing to offer a recommendation and not providing appropriate guidance would violate the duties of beneficence and nonmaleficence by leaving either the patient or surrogate decision-maker to carry the burden of making complex medical decisions without professional counsel.[31]

As shared decision-making is designed to integrate patients' self-determination with medical expertise, the process should include the freedom to ignore certain individual aspects of the process. In other words, shared decision-making does not preclude a patient's choosing a more physician-directed process, as long as the patient is fully informed. Studies of patient preference have found that the most significant differences in preference center around the proportion of value associated with a choice. For example, 55% of respondents in one study reported preferring to have control over value-laden decisions, whereas 40% wished to share control equally and 5% wanted their doctors to make value-laden decisions on their behalf. The study also found that patients tended to prefer for their physicians to make technical decisions.[32] Another study of 13,902 patients at the University of Chicago found that 71.1% wished to delegate the majority of their decisions to the clinician.[33]

WHEN DISPUTES REMAIN AND SPECIALIST SUPPORT IS NEEDED

Despite effective shared decision-making, conflicts between decision-makers and care teams remain a feature of end-of-life care, and resolution can be difficult.[34] Palliative care teams are often formally involved when such tension occurs. Whereas many palliative care consults involve pain management or other symptom control, patients with neurologic illness who receive inpatient palliative care consultation typically have more severe illness and consults are more likely to be requested for assistance in defining goals of care or deciding about withdrawal of life-sustaining treatments.[35] Among the specific challenges identified for patients hospitalized with neurologic diagnoses is highly variable prognostication.[36] This challenge includes not only predicting survival but also predicting long-term neurologic recovery, as surrogate decision makers most often make decisions regarding survival without reliably knowing what future quality of life will be.[37]

SOCIAL SCIENCE EFFORTS TO IMPROVE SHARED DECISION-MAKING

Efforts to identify and understand barriers to effective shared decision-making and dispute resolution are particularly important in neurology. Studies on neurologic prognostication have found that physicians tend to be overly optimistic about survival and quality of life; however, there are also obvious concerns that pessimism could lead to self-fulfilling prophecies or therapeutic nihilism.[38] A large variability in end-of-life decision-making has also been observed between centers. Rates of withdrawal of life-sustaining treatment after stroke can range from 0% to 96% between centers after adjusting for disease severity and age.[39] One study examining clinician–family meetings regarding plans for critically ill neurologic patients found that clinicians' prognostic communication was highly variable, especially with regard to eliciting the patient's or family's values and preferences.[40] Elicitation rather than assumption of values is particularly important in the ICU, as the physician's perception that a patient would not want life support has been identified as an independent predictor of ventilator support being withdrawn.[41]

Formal models have been proposed to standardize clinician's prognostication and related communication, including the *Anticipating-Anchoring-Tailoring-Debiasing* approach, which is specific to patients with advanced neurologic disease. This approach emphasizes anticipating the types of prognostic information that will be most meaningful during the encounter with importance placed on "how long" and "how well." The approach then encourages clinicians to anchor individual patients to data-driven trajectories or survival ranges and tailor prognosis to the individual's patient-specific data and trajectory. Debiasing then focuses on acknowledging both personal and system level biases in an effort to overcome inappropriate influences.[38]

Well-known conversation tools, including REMAP, NURSE, ask-tell-ask, and "tell me more" can also help physicians promote shared decision-making.[42,43] Many institutions also use formalized, commercial communications resources to provide clinicians evidence-based training on communication in serious illness. These workshops have been found effective in both palliative and non-palliative training programs in English and in other languages.[44,45]

PATIENT EDUCATION AND DECISION-MAKING TOOLS

Patient facing decision-making aids provide another opportunity to standardize the approach to shared decision-making. One of the more widely applicable decision-making aids is the "Best Case/Worst Case" communication tool, which was originally developed for acute surgical decision-making, but it is also intended for use with difficult treatment decisions for frail adults. This tool uses a written diagram to illustrate likely outcomes from an intervention and prompts the provider to elicit the patient's or family's values and encourages discussion and deliberation.[46]

The LEAD Guide (Life Planning in Early Alzheimer's and Dementia) is a decision-making aid developed and validated in end-of-life planning for patients with, or who are at risk of, Alzheimer's disease and related dementias. The LEAD Guide is designed to be used both independently by families and in the clinical setting to elicit patients' preferences and values and to empower surrogate decision makers to assume responsibility when a patient becomes incapacitated. This initiative was motivated in part by concerns that the scope of typical advanced directives is limited, leading patients to rely on orally expressed wishes and on the assumption that their loved ones would know what they want at the end of life.[47]

A decision-making aid was also created for surrogate decision makers participating in meetings about goals-of-care decisions for patients after severe acute brain injury, including hemispheric acute ischemic infarct, intracerebral hemorrhage, or traumatic brain injury. Muehlschlegel and colleagues piloted a decision aid provided to surrogates before clinician–family meetings that help family members identify their loved one's values. The use of this decision aid was found to be feasible and was well received by family members.[48] Similarly, a comprehensive education and decision-making tool specific to ischemic and hemorrhagic stroke has undergone initial clinical studies.[49]

TIME-LIMITED TRIALS

Ultimately, when consensus about appropriate end-of-life care cannot be reached, time-limited trials of intervention can provide a way forward. Before offering a time-limited trial, all members of the care team should agree on treatment options and prognosis, and this consensus should be communicated to either the patient or surrogate decision maker with the goal of clarifying values and priorities. To be effective, a time-limited trial must include a well-defined treatment plan and time frame for reevaluation that includes markers of both deterioration and improvement that are ideally linked to visible signs for decision makers. Before initiation of the trial, all parties should agree on what may be done when it is time to reevaluate outcomes.[50]

When offered in appropriate situations, time-limited trials can build rapport between families and the care team by allowing families to understand risks and benefits of potential treatments and observe the natural course of disease processes.[50] Establishing clearly defined goals promotes the success of a time-limited trial. Such an approach may also be more straightforward in the care of patients with few confounding variables, such as single-organ failure.[51] Time-limited trials can also allow collection of longitudinal data if either prognosis is unclear or there is disagreement among the care team.[52]

TREATMENT OF FAMILY MEMBER DISTRESS

Complicated grief and even post-traumatic stress disorder (PTSD) have been demonstrated at significant rates among caregivers of patients in neurocritical care units for whom treatment decisions are difficult.[53] Similarly, surrogates of patients with severe acute brain injury on prolonged mechanical ventilation have persistently elevated anxiety and depression symptoms compared with surrogates of those on ventilation for other conditions.[54] Formal efforts to study and improve outcomes for caregivers and surrogate decision-makers have focused on communication. Wendler and colleagues argued that improving communication can decrease the emotional burden of shared decision-making.[55] Specific communication strategies that have been proposed to reduce caregiver burden include building trust with family by meeting soon after admission, designating a consistent member of the care team to lead conversations, and—if the focus of treatment shifts from recovery to palliation—avoiding such phrases as "withdrawal of care" and focusing instead on the ways in which the medical team will continue to provide care to the patient.[56]

In addition to the primary care team, resources such as chaplaincy and spiritual care can often support the family's or surrogate's ability to cope. A randomized clinical trial showed that surrogates with scheduled, semi-structured visits from a chaplain had significantly improved levels of anxiety at follow-up.[57] Chaplains can also assist in determining how a patient's spiritual beliefs might affect preferences for care. Particularly when a patient of family has strong religious beliefs or cultural traditions around medical care and end-of-life, ignoring spiritual and cultural needs is a detriment to the patient and family and may harm their relationship with the care team.

RECOGNITION OF THE IMPACT OF MORAL DISTRESS

Attempts to improve the partnership between patient and clinician that focus on maximizing the patient's self-determination balanced with clinician advocacy will inevitably be imperfect. Because perspectives on what is most biologically plausible and most consistent with the patient's values will inherently differ, some patients will desire a care path that is not consistent with what a clinician would consider either medically advisable or ethically appropriate. This discrepancy will often cause a measure of distress to members of the clinical team, which in recent times has been identified as "moral distress." In the past, such stress was considered the result of the violation of the professional's "moral integrity" or "physician autonomy," but the more contemporary term moral distress recognized the emotional impact without qualifying whether the distress is inherently justified. Philosopher Andrew Jameton first used the term in 1984, defining it as, "knowing what to do in an ethical situation but not being allowed to do it."[58] Those experiencing moral distress feel a sense of powerlessness caused by internal or external restrictions, whether actual or perceived. The nursing profession has been on forefront of recognizing the impact of moral distress. The American Association of Critical Care Nurses offered formal guidance on the importance of recognizing the impact of moral distress and affirmed the importance of self-care and plans to mitigate the impact in "The 4A's to Rise Above Moral Distress."[59] Elizabeth Epstein and Ann Hamric, two thought leaders on this topic, explored the impact of unresolved moral distress, which they labeled "moral residue," and identified an accumulation of unresolved moral distress as "the crescendo effect."[60]

Moral distress has been explored among many health care groups, including neurology trainees. A mixed methods study in Germany that included 107 neurology residents found that 96.3% of the respondents experienced moral distress weekly, related to insufficient time, errors, difficulty meeting expectations, legal fears, incentive programs, and administrative tasks. Forty-three percent reported considering leaving the field and 65.4% indicated that they wanted more support.[61] The identification of multiple causes of moral distress does raise the question of how often these stresses truly involve violations of moral principles, but if a stress has the potential to affect patient care and fulfillment of the physician's duties, then indeed a wide range of stresses can be considered moral distress.

Moral distress has also received attention in the mental health community and the military, which has expanded the term to "moral injury" in cases of where the experience has a profound impact. One review of the topic that included 116 empirical studies of moral injury in military scenarios indicated that attention to traditional treatment for PTSD may not be adequate to address the moral component of the injury, which may require something akin to "moral repair."[62] The recognition of moral distress and its relationship to combat burnout has let to numerous attempts to mitigate the impact with more than 20 studies testing the effectiveness of interventions, most commonly education-based.[63]

SUMMARY

Balancing effective medical treatment with a patient's goals of care has become increasingly complex as advanced medical technology offers a still incomplete ability to improve health in a way that the patient may or may not be able to appreciate. We can neither maintain a physician directed decision-making strategy nor offer patients a menu of options and expect them to understand the consequences of their medical decisions. Developing a robust patient–physician partnership committed to communication that elicits values and goals of care is a necessary part of practicing standard-of-care medicine. The challenge moving forward will be how to create the space and time to execute this process and offer adequate sources of information to optimize patient engagement.

CLINICS CARE POINTS

- Always begin with an assessment of the patient's understanding of their disease. They will not be able to make decisions regarding care if they don't first understand their pathology.

- Build a partnership with your patient so they understand the complex medical and value-laden nature of medical decision-making.
- Offering only the options you want a patient to choose is not offering them a choice.
- Utilize additional resources in cases of disagreement over direction of care.

DISCLOSURE

The authors have no relevant disclosures or conflicts of interest.

REFERENCES

1. Lloyd GER, editor. Hippocratic writings. London: Penguin Group; 1983.
2. Jones WHS. In: trans. Hippocrates, the Art. Cambridge MA: Harvard University Press; 1923. reprinted in SR Reiser, AJ Dyke, WJ Curran, eds Ethics in Medicine: Historical Perspectives and Contemporary Concerns. Cambridge, MA: MIT Press, 1977: 5-9.
3. Kienle GS, Kiene H. Clinical judgement and the medical profession. J Eval Clin Pract 2011;17:621–7.
4. Heitman E. Ethical issues in technology assessment: conceptual categories and procedural considerations. Intl J Technol Assess Health Care 1998;14:544–66.
5. Cassell EJ. Dying in a technological society. Hastings Cent Stud 1974;2(2):31–6.
6. Kubler-Ross E. On death and dying. New York: Macmillan Publishing Co; 1969.
7. Fuchs VR. The growing demand for medical care. N Engl J Med 1968;279:190–5.
8. Brett AS, McCullough LB. When patients request specific interventions: defining the limits of the physician's obligation. N Engl J Med 1986;315:1347–51.
9. Sabatino CP. The evolution of health care advance planning law and policy. Milbank Q 2010;88(2):211–39.
10. Meisel A. The legal consensus about forgoing life-sustaining treatment: its status and its prospects. Kennedy Inst Ethics J 1992;2(4):309–45.
11. Schneiderman LJ, Jecker NS, Jonsen AR. Medical futility: its meaning and ethical implications. Ann Intern Med 1990;112:949–54.
12. American Medical Association. Council on Ethical and Judicial Affairs. Medical futility in end-of-life care: report of the Council on Ethical and Judicial Affairs. JAMA 1999;281:937–41.
13. Schneiderman LJ. Defining medical futility and improving medical care. J bioeth Inq 2011;123:123–31.
14. Brody BA, Halevy A. Is futility a futile concept? J Med Philos 1995;20:123–44.
15. Halevy A, Brody BA for the Houston City-Wide Taskforce on Medical Futility. A multi-institution collaborative policy on medical futility. JAMA 1996;276:571–4.
16. Bosslet GT, Pope TM, Rubenfeld GD, et al. An Official ATS/AACN/ACCP/ESICM/SCCM Policy Statement: Responding to Requests for Potentially Inappropriate Treatments in Intensive Care Units. Am J Respir Crit Care Med 2015;191(11):1318–30.
17. Timmermans S. The Engaged Patient: The Relevance of Patient-Physician Communication for Twenty-First-Century Health. J Health Soc Behav 2020;61(3):259–73.
18. Taylor Keith. Paternalism, participation and partnership – The evolution of patient centeredness in the consultation. Patient Educ Couns 2009;74:150–5.
19. National Commission for the Protection of Human Subjects of Biomedical and Behavioral Research. The Belmont report: Ethical principles and guidelines for

the protection of human subjects of research. U.S. Department of Health and Human Services, 1979 Available at: https://www.hhs.gov/ohrp/regulations-and-policy/belmont-report/read-the-belmont-report/index.html/. Accessed May 9, 2023.

20. Beauchamp TL, Childress J. Principles of biomedical ethics. New York: Oxford University Press; 1979.

21. Robinson JH, Callister LC, Berry JA, et al. Patient-centered care and adherence: definitions and applications to improve outcomes. J Am Acad Nurse Pract 2008; 20:600–7.

22. Khan MW, Muehlschlegel S. Shared Decision Making in Neurocritical Care. Neurol Clin 2017;35:825–34.

23. Gampel E. Does professional autonomy protect medical futility judgments? Bioethics 2006;20(2):92–104.

24. Swenson SL, Buell S, Zettler P, et al. Patient-centered communication: do patients really prefer it? J Gen Intern Med 2004;19:1069–79.

25. Leonard LD, Cumbler E, Schulick R, et al. From paternalistic to patient-centered: strategies to support patients with the immediate release of medical records. Am J Surg 2021;222:909–10.

26. Colligan E, Metzler A, Tiryak E. Shared decision-making in multiple sclerosis. Mult Scler 2017;23(2):185–90.

27. Pickrell WO, Elwyn G, Smith PEM. Shared decision-making in epilepsy management. Epilepsy Behav 2015;47:78–82.

28. Corell A, Guo A, Vecchio TG, et al. Shared decision-making in neurosurgery: a scoping review. Acta Neurochir 2021;163:2371–81.

29. Rubin MA. The collaborative autonomy model of medical decision-making. Neurocritical Care 2014;20(2):311–8.

30. Bomhof-Roordink H. Key components of shared decision-making models: a systematic review. BMJ Open 2019;9(12):e031763.

31. Cai X, Robinson J, Muehlschlegel S, et al. Patient preference and surrogate decision making in neuroscience intensive care units. Neurocritical Care 2015; 23(1):131–41.

32. Johnson SK, Bautista CA, Hong SY, et al. An empirical study of surrogates' preferred level of control over value-laden life support decisions in intensive care units. Am J Respir Crit Care Med 2011;183:915–21.

33. Ruhnke GW, Tak HJ, Meltzer DO. Association of preferences for participation in decision-making with care satisfaction among hospitalized patients. JAMA Netw Open 2020;3(10):e2018766.

34. Burt RA. The medical futility debate: patient choice, physician obligation, and end-of-life care. J Palliat Med 2002;5(2):249–54.

35. Taylor BL, O'Riordan DL, Pantilat SZ, et al. Inpatients with neurologic disease referred for palliative care consultation. Neurology 2019;92(17):e1975–81.

36. Sloane K.L., Miller J.J., Piquet A., et al., Prognostication in Acute Neurological Emergencies, J Stroke Cerebrovasc Dis, 31 (3), 2022, 106277.

37. Goss AL, Creutzfeldt CJ. Neuropalliative Care in the Inpatient Setting. Semin Neurol 2021;41(5):619–30.

38. Holloway RG, Gramling R, Kelly AG. Estimating and communicating prognosis in advanced neurologic disease. Neurology 2013;80(8):764–72.

39. Holloway RG, Benesch CG, Burgin WS, et al. Prognosis and decision making in severe stroke. JAMA 2005;294(6):725–33.

40. Ge C, Godd AL, Crawford S, et al. Variability of prognostic communication in critically ill neurologic patients: a pilot multicenter mixed-methods study. Critical Care Explorer 2022;4(2):e0640.

41. Cook D, Rocker G, Marshall J, et al. Withdrawal of mechanical ventilation in anticipation of death in the intensive care unit. N Engl J Med 2003;349(12):1123–32.

42. Back AL, Arnold RM, Baile WF, et al. Approaching difficult communication tasks in oncology. CA Cancer J Clin 2005;55(3):164–77.

43. Childers JW, Back AL, Tulsky JA, et al. REMAP: A framework for goals of Care Conversations. J Oncol Pract 2017;13(10):e844–50.

44. Lockwood BJ, Gustin J, Verbeck N, et al. Training to promote empathic communication in graduate medical education: a shared learning intervention in internal medicine and general surgery. Palliat Med Rep 2022;3(1):26–35.

45. Ito K, Uemura T, Yuasa M, et al. The feasibility of virtual VitalTalk workshops in Japanese: can faculty members in the US effectively teach communication skills virtually to learners in Japan? Am J Hosp Palliat Care 2022;39(7):785–90.

46. Kruser JM, Nabozny MJ, Steffense NM, et al. Best case/worst case": qualitative evaluation of a novel communication tool for difficult in-the-moment surgical decisions. J Am Geriatr Soc 2015;63(9):1805–11.

47. Dassel K, et al. Development of a dementia-focused end-of-life planning tool: The LEAD Guide (Life-Planning in Early Alzheimer's and Dementia). Innovations Aging 2019;3(3):igz024.

48. Muehlschlegel S, Goostrey K, Flahive J, et al. A pilot randomized clinical trial of a goals-of-care decision aid for surrogates of severe acute brain injury patients. Neurology 2022;99(14):e1446–55.

49. Chen EP, Arslanian-Engoren C, Newhouse W, et al. Development and usability testing of Understanding Stroke, a tailored life-sustaining treatment decision support tool for stroke surrogate decision makers. BMC Palliat Care 2020;19(1):110.

50. Quill TE, Holloway R. Time-limited trials near the end of life. JAMA 2011;306(13):1483–4.

51. Bruce CR, Liane C, Blumenthal-Barby JS, et al. Barriers and facilitators to initiating and completing time-limited trials in critical care. Crit Care Med 2015;43(12):2535–43.

52. Beil M, Sviri S, Flatten H, et al. On predictions in critical care: The individual prognostication fallacy in elderly patients. J Crit Care 2021;61:34–8.

53. Trevick SA, Lord AS. Post-traumatic stress disorder and complicated grief are common in caregivers of neuro-ICU patients. Neurocritical Care 2017;26(3):436–43.

54. Wendlandt B, Olm-Shimpan C, Ceppe A, et al. Surrogates of patients with severe acute brain injury experience persistent anxiety and depression over the 6 months after ICU admission. J Pain Symptom Manag 2022;63(6):e633–9.

55. Wendler D, Rid A. Systematic review: the effect on surrogates of making treatment decisions for others. Ann Intern Med 2011;154(5):336–46.

56. Rath KA, Tucker KL, Lewis A. Fluctuating code status: strategies to minimize end-of-life conflict in the neurocritical care setting. Am J Hosp Palliat Care 2022;39(1):79–85.

57. Torke AM, et al. Effects of spiritual care on well-being of intensive care family surrogates: a clinical trial. J Pain Symptom Manage 2022;S0885–3924.

58. Savel RH, Munro CL. Moral distress, moral courage. Am J Crit Care 2015;24(4):276–8.

59. American Association of Critical Care Nurses. The 4A's to rise above moral distress. Available at: https://www.emergingrnleader.com/wp-content/uploads/2012/06/4As_to_Rise_Above_Moral_Distress.pdf Accessed March 14, 2023.

60. Epstein EG, Hamric AB. Moral distress, moral residue, and the crescendo effect. J Clin Ethics 2009;20(4):330–42.

61. Hildesheim H, et al. Moral distress among residents in neurology: a pilot study. Neurol Res Pract 2021;3(6):1–9.

62. Griffin BJ. Moral injury: an integrative review. J Trauma Stress 2019;32:250–362.

63. Amos VK, Epstein E. Moral distress interventions: an integrative literature review. Nurs Ethics 2022;29(3):582–607.

Brain Death
Ethical and Legal Challenges

Danielle Feng, MD[a], Ariane Lewis, MD[b,c],*

KEYWORDS

- Brain death • Ethics • Family • Legal • UDDA • Uniform Determination of Death Act

KEY POINTS

- Brain death/death by neurologic criteria is considered legal death throughout the United States and much of the world, but it remains a source of ethical and legal controversy
- Although objections to brain death/death by neurologic criteria are usually based on religious beliefs, views vary both within and among religions
- Public understanding and acceptance of brain death/death by neurologic criteria is poor and this is in part due to inaccurate portrayals in the media, television, and movies
- United States courts have issued different decisions about the management of objections to brain death/death by neurologic criteria, but decisions in the United Kingdom courts have been more consistent
- The Uniform Determination of Death Act, a recommended statute in the United States that equates death by circulatory-respiratory criteria and brain death/death by neurologic criteria, may be revised

HISTORY OF BRAIN DEATH/DEATH BY NEUROLOGIC CRITERIA

The advent of defibrillators[1] and ventilators[2] resulted in the ability to sustain circulatory-respiratory and other systemic functions in patients with irreversible loss of brain function, a state first described in 1959 by Mollaret and Goulon as "le coma depassé" or "a state beyond coma."[3] This new clinical reality led to an ethical quandary: continuation of circulatory-respiratory support was recognized to be futile, but while some clinicians considered this state to be equivalent to death by circulatory-respiratory criteria, others thought that it was morally wrong to withhold treatment.[3] The status of these individuals was discussed by international medical consortia, including the World Health

Funding: No authors received funding for their work on this article.
[a] Department of Neurology, Harbor-UCLA Medical Center, 1000 West Carson Street, Torrance, CA 90502, USA; [b] Department of Neurology, NYU Langone Medical Center, 530 First Avenue, Skirball-7R, New York, NY 10016, USA; [c] Department of Neurosurgery, NYU Langone Medical Center, 530 First Avenue, Skirball-7R, New York, NY 10016, USA
* Corresponding author. Department of Neurology, NYU Langone Medical Center, 530 First Avenue, Skirball-7R, New York, NY 10016.
E-mail address: ariane.kansas.lewis@gmail.com

Organization and World Medical Association,[4] further fueling the need for ethical and legal consensus about the implications of this state.

In 1968, a multidisciplinary ad hoc committee led by Dr. Henry Beecher, the Chair of Anesthesiology at Harvard Medical School, introduced conditions for the determination of brain death/death by neurologic criteria (BD/DNC) in a landmark article entitled "A Definition of Irreversible Coma."[5] These criteria included clinical observations of (1) unreceptivity and unresponsivity, (2) no movements or breathing, and (3) no reflexes; use of an electroencephalogram (EEG), if available, was encouraged. At this time, organ transplantation and resuscitative efforts in intensive care units were in their infancy, and Beecher argued against the continuation of organ support for "hopelessly unconscious" patients.[6] The committee thought that the medical community was ready to adopt a new means to determine death (via neurologic criteria) and that neurologic death would be seamlessly accepted as legal death. The committee also thought that no statutory changes would be needed unless debate surfaced about use of neurologic criteria to declare death.

Although valiant in its intent to establish an expanded definition of death, the article was considered controversial for several reasons. The argument that "irreversible coma" was equivalent to death met some resistance medically, legally, and socially, and there was confusion about the clinical conditions described by the committee.[7,8] Further, the concept that BD/DNC required loss of whole brain function differed from the United Kingdom's Conference of Medical Royal Colleges view that it only required loss of brainstem function.[9] As such, a patient with catastrophic infratentorial brain injury who had electrical activity on EEG could be deemed deceased in the United Kingdom, but alive in the United States.[10]

In 1979, President Jimmy Carter formed the Commission for the Study of Ethical Problems in Medicine and Biomedical and Behavioral Research, for which one objective was to define death. Members of the Commission, who had backgrounds in law, sociology, medicine, ethics, and health economics,[11] carefully reviewed the concept of BD/DNC and met with physicians, philosophers, religious officials, ethicists, and representatives of the American Bar Association, American Medical Association, and the National Conference of Commissioners on Uniform State Laws. They also reviewed legal language on death from around the country, noting that BD/DNC was accepted as death in 27 states. In 1981, in a report entitled "Defining Death: Medical, Legal, and Ethical Issues in the Determination of Death," the Commission published the Uniform Determination of Death Act (UDDA), which states that "[a]n individual who has sustained either (1) irreversible cessation of circulatory and respiratory functions, or (2) irreversible cessation of all functions of the entire brain, including the brain stem, is dead. A determination of death must be made in accordance with accepted medical standards."[12]

In the ensuing years, every state accepted BD/DNC as the legal equivalent of death by circulatory-respiratory criteria.[13] Death is defined statutorily in most states, except Illinois and Washington, where the UDDA was adopted judicially, and New York, where death is described in rules and regulations. The complete language of the UDDA is used by 71% of states (variations are described in **Table 1**).[13]

To further clarify the process for the determination of BD/DNC, guidelines were published for (1) children in 1987, then updated in 2011 by the Society of Critical Care Medicine, American Academy of Pediatrics, and Child Neurology Society[14,15] and (2) adults in 1995, then updated in 2010 by the American Academy of Neurology (AAN).[16,17] These guidelines describe the following aspects of the determination of BD/DNC: (1) the prerequisites (including exclusion of confounders or mimics), (2) the clinical evaluation to assess for coma and brainstem areflexia, (3) the performance

Table 1
Variations in state definitions of death compared with the Uniform Determination of Death Act

States that do not use "irreversible cessation of circulatory and respiratory functions" (2/51 states)	Arizona, North Carolina
States that do not use ""irreversible cessation of all functions of the entire brain, including the brain stem" (6/51 states)	Arizona, Illinois, Iowa, Louisiana, North Carolina
States that do not use "determination of death must be made in accordance with accepted medical standards" (14/51 states)	Florida, New Jersey: "in accordance with currently accepted medical standards" Georgia: does not include "medical standards" Hawaii: "based on ordinary standards of current medical practice" Illinois, Kentucky, Missouri: "usual and customary standards of medical practice" Iowa, Maryland, Texas, Virginia: "ordinary standards of medical practice" Louisiana: "ordinary standards of approved medical practice" Minnesota: "generally accepted medical standards" North Carolina: "ordinary and accepted standards"

Based on data from Lewis A, Cahn-Fuller K, Caplan A. Shouldn't Dead Be Dead?: The Search for a Uniform Definition of Death. Journal of Law, Medicine & Ethics. 2017;45(1):112-128.

of an apnea test to evaluate for inability to breathe spontaneously in the setting of elevated blood levels of carbon dioxide, and (4) the use of ancillary testing if the full clinical evaluation cannot be completed (such as in the setting of facial trauma). At present, the AAN is collaborating with adult and pediatric BD/DNC experts to develop a singular consensus practice guideline on determination of BD/DNC for persons of all ages.[18] Additionally, the AAN endorsed that death has occurred when there is irreversible loss of all functions of the entire brain, including the brainstem, as demonstrated by complete loss of consciousness (coma), brainstem reflexes, and the independent capacity to breathe, in the absence of any factors that imply reversibility.[19]

Finally, the equivalence of a declaration of BD/DNC to a declaration of death by circulatory-respiratory criteria was embraced by 5 world federations and 30 international, national, and regional medical societies with the publication of the World Brain Death Project in 2020.[20] National policies on the determination of BD/DNC exist throughout much of Asia, Australia, Europe, North America, and South America.[21]

WHY DO SOME PEOPLE OBJECT TO BRAIN DEATH/DEATH BY NEUROLOGIC CRITERIA?

The public's understanding and acceptance of BD/DNC, however, has largely lagged behind the medicolegal community.[22] A review of 24 empirical studies on public understanding and acceptance of BD/DNC demonstrated many people (1) have never heard of BD/DNC, (2) thought it is possible to recover from BD/DNC, (3) do not think BD/DNC is legal death, and (4) would not consent to organ donation after BD/DNC.[21,23-27]

Families object to BD/DNC for several reasons, but objections are often attributed to religious beliefs, although religious and cultural views about the determination of death vary both between and within faiths (**Table 2**).[28,29] For example, Pope John Paul II accepted BD/DNC as death,[30] but a survey of hospital chaplains in the United States[31,32] found that objections to BD/DNC were predominantly made by families of Evangelical Protestant and Catholic patients (results were not adjusted based on the overall number of patients who practiced a given religion). This demonstrates that individual, rather than institutional, ethics can play a role in religious objections to BD/DNC. The study further found that of the 521 chaplains surveyed, 84% equated BD/DNC with death by circulatory-respiratory criteria, and only a minority thought that a patient's family should be able to decide whether (1) an evaluation for the determination of BD/DNC is performed (16%) or (2) organ support should be discontinued after determination of BD/DNC (30%). Similarly, a survey of Muslim health professionals in the United States found that 84% of respondents considered BD/DNC to be equivalent to death by circulatory-respiratory criteria, but only 33% thought that most Muslims would share this belief.[33] However, 50% of respondents thought that a patient's family should be able to decide whether an evaluation for the determination of BD/DNC is performed, and 48% of respondents believed that a patient's family should be able to decide whether organ support should be discontinued after determination of BD/DNC. Additionally, a survey of rabbis found that 78% of respondents considered BD/DNC to be death.[32]

Objections to BD/DNC are also made for nonreligious reasons including the (1) belief that death only occurs when the heart stops beating, (2) belief in the potential for recovery/miracles, (3) fear that determination of BD/DNC may be inaccurate, (4) concern that determination of BD/DNC is motivated by a desire for organ procurement, or (5) hope for personal financial gain including the desire to continue receiving social security benefits.[23,28,29] https://paperpile.com/c/4YAgSn/LHay These objections may be fueled, in part, by inaccurate portrayals of BD/DNC in the media, which can lead to a lack of understanding of the distinction between BD/DNC and disorders of consciousness and raise doubts about the validity of a determination of BD/DNC.[22,24–27]

HOW DO CLINICIANS HANDLE OBJECTIONS TO BRAIN DEATH/DEATH BY NEUROLOGIC CRITERIA?

Surveys of clinicians involved in the determination of BD/DNC in the United States and Canada demonstrated that management of objections to BD/DNC is inconsistent.[29,34] Views varied about what medical treatments respondents were willing to either continue or initiate after determination of BD/DNC (eg, antibiotics, vasopressors, nutrition, and intravenous fluids). However, respondents rarely discontinued organ support after determination of BD/DNC when a family objected.[34] Reasons to continue organ support included fear of negative media coverage, litigation, or upsetting the family.[28]

Strategies to address objections to BD/DNC vary across hospitals, and a review of 330 United States hospital policies on BD/DNC found that 75% do not address management of objections.[28] Of the policies that provide guidance about how to manage these objections, recommendations differed (**Fig. 1**).

WHAT HAPPENS WHEN OBJECTIONS TO BRAIN DEATH/DEATH BY NEUROLOGIC CRITERIA ARE BROUGHT TO COURT?

If hospitals are unable to resolve controversies with families about determination of BD/DNC or discontinuation of organ support after BD/DNC, these disputes are

Table 2
An overview of beliefs about death across religions

Religion	Beliefs About Death
Buddhism	The Buddhist cannon texts include the Tripitaka, Mahayana Sutras, and the Tibetan Book of the Dead. There is no consensus regarding criteria for death. Followers think life and death are a continuum and the spirit continues after death. Buddhists think that *death occurs when the spirit, vitality, heat, and sentience of the individual leave the body,* which is difficult to define medically. However, the overarching tenants of Buddhism are altruism and elimination of suffering. As such, although followers may not accept BD/DNC, they may favor discontinuation of organ support in a patient with a catastrophic brain injury to minimize suffering[49–51]
Catholicism	Jus Canonicum, the Catholic legal system, is based on sources divided into "Sources of Being" and "Sources of Knowing," which include both historical and contemporary religious figures (ie, Jesus Christ, the Apostles, Holy Bible, popes, bishops, and so forth). *Death is defined as the separation of the soul and body,* but the departure of the soul is difficult to define medically. In an address in 2000, Pope John Paul II proposed that medical professionals are responsible for determining loss of an individual organism's "integrative capacity." He stated that "therefore, a health-worker professionally responsible for ascertaining death can use these [neurological] criteria in each individual case as the basis for arriving at that degree of assurance in ethical judgement which moral teaching describes as 'moral certainty' [in the fact of death]," and that "with regard to the parameters used today for ascertaining death - whether the 'encephalic' signs or the more traditional cardio-respiratory signs - the Church does not make technical decisions." However, subsequent Catholic commentary demonstrates that the religion's views on BD/DNC are unsettled.[52–55]
Hinduism	Hindu followers think that *the soul has neither beginning nor end and is reincarnated by taking on another physical body, so death is simply a series of changes between bodies.* Current Hindu philosophy defines "brain death" as the loss of "higher brain function," but BD/DNC is not generally accepted.[56–58]
Islam	Islamic Law is based on the Holy Quran, Sunnah, Ijma' and Qiyas. *Death is defined as the departure of the soul from the body,* but there is no consensus about when this occurs. Scholars and fatwa differ in their legal opinions on BD/DNC. It is accepted by the Islamic Medical Association of North America, Islamic Fiqh Academic of the Organization of the Islamic Conference, and the Muslim World League but a minority of organizations only accepts death by circulatory-respiratory criteria. However, despite discord about whether BD/DNC is indeed death, most Islamic jurists agree that it is religiously permissible to withdraw organ support after the determination of BD/DNC[59,60]
Judaism	Halakhah, the Jewish legal system, is based on the Torah, rabbinic law, various historical authorities, and traditional customs. *Death is defined as the departure of the soul from the body, but there is disagreement about whether it should be identified by irreversible cessation of spontaneous respiration or irreversible cessation of vital motion (any spontaneous movement that contributes to the biological viability of the organism).*[61–64]
Shinto	Shintoism does not have a set of laws, but encourages its followers to live in harmony with nature, in accordance with deities of nature known as kami. After death, the spirit lives on with the living and can become kami. There

(continued on next page)

Table 2 (continued)	
Religion	**Beliefs About Death**
	is *no official consensus regarding death, but because Japanese society has generally been resistant to organ donation (due to an emphasis on the need for an intact body for funeral rites), which is culturally intertwined with the determination of BD/DNC, BD/DNC is not widely accepted.*[65,66]

brought to court. Although most legal disputes about BD/DNC occur in the United States, cases have also been brought to court in Canada and the United Kingdom (**Table 3**).[20,35] In the United States, the decisions in these cases vary because every state has their own legal system. For example, when two families objected to performance of an evaluation for determination of BD/DNC, a court in Montana ruled that the evaluation could not be completed but a court in Virginia ruled that the evaluation could proceed.[36] Contrastingly, judges in the United Kingdom routinely reference decisions from earlier court cases about objections to BD/DNC and consistently rule against accommodation of these objections.[35]

SHOULD CONSENT BE REQUIRED BEFORE PERFORMING AN EVALUATION FOR THE DETERMINATION OF BRAIN DEATH/DEATH BY NEUROLOGIC CRITERIA?

One way to address objections to BD/DNC would be to require consent for the evaluation. In general, a basic ethical principle of medical practice is that clinicians should obtain consent before performing a procedure. Of course, there are notable exceptions, such as in cases of life-threatening emergencies where no decision-maker is present. Survey data demonstrated that three-quarters of physicians involved in the determination of BD/DNC did not think consent should be required.[23,34]

Arguments in favor of obtaining consent to perform an evaluation for the determination of BD/DNC center around respect for autonomy, freedom of religion, lack of direct benefit to the patient, concern about possible harm during the apnea test, and distrust of the validity of the evaluation.[37–39] Multiple arguments are raised against obtaining

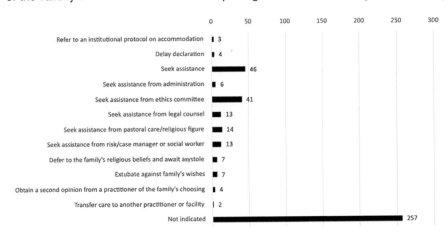

Fig. 1. United States hospital protocol guidance about the management of objections to brain death/death by neurologic criteria (n = 330). (*Based on data from* Lewis A, Varelas P, Greer D. Prolonging Support After Brain Death: When Families Ask for More. Neurocrit Care. 2016;24(3):481-487. https://doi.org/10.1007/s12028-015-0209-7)

Table 3
A few recent objections to brain death/death by neurologic criteria that were brought to court

Jahi McMath (California, USA)[67,68] 2013	McMath was a 13-year-old girl who developed hypoxic-ischemic brain injury secondary to hemorrhage following a tonsillectomy. She was declared brain dead/dead by neurologic criteria, but when her family objected to discontinuation of organ support, the court allowed her family to transfer her to New Jersey (where death is not declared by neurologic criteria in the setting of a religious objection) and organ support was continued until circulatory-respiratory arrest in 2017.
Aden Hailu (Nevada, USA)[13,69] 2015	Hailu was a 20-year-old woman who developed hypoxic-ischemic brain injury during an appendectomy. She was declared brain dead/dead by neurologic criteria, but her father objected to the declaration. The county court granted permission for the hospital to discontinue organ support, but the Nevada Supreme Court decided the evaluation for the determination of death by neurologic criteria, which was done in accordance with the 2010 AAN guideline, was not performed in accordance with "accepted medical standards" because there was no EEG evidence of BD/DNC. Her heart subsequently stopped, but Nevada updated their legal definition of death to specify that the AAN guideline is considered the accepted medical standard for declaration of BD/DNC in adults.
Allen Callaway (Montana, USA)[36] 2016	Callaway was a 6-year-old boy who had hypoxic-ischemic brain injury after drowning. The hospital planned to perform an evaluation for the determination of BD/DNC, but his mother objected to the apnea test. The court ruled that the hospital could not perform the evaluation without parental consent.
Mirranda Grace Lawson (Virginia, USA)[36] 2016	Lawson was a 2-year-old girl who had hypoxic-ischemic brain injury after choking. The hospital planned to perform an evaluation for determination of BD/DNC, but her parents objected to the apnea test. The court ruled that the hospital could perform the evaluation, but her parents appealed the decision and she had a circulatory-respiratory arrest before completion of the appeal process, so the appeal was withdrawn.
Israel Stinson (California, USA)[70] 2016	Stinson was a 2-year-old boy who had hypoxic-ischemic brain injury after an asthma attack led to a cardiac arrest. He was declared brain dead/dead by neurologic criteria, but his mother objected to discontinuation of organ support and a judge allowed her to transfer him to Guatemala. However, she subsequently brought him to Children's Hospital in Los Angeles and a court allowed the hospital to discontinue organ support.
Taquisha McKitty (Ontario, Canada)[71] 2018	McKitty was a 27-year-old woman who had hypoxic-ischemic brain injury due to a cardiac arrest in the setting of a drug overdose. She was declared brain dead/dead by neurologic criteria, but her family objected to discontinuation of organ support based on their religious beliefs. The Ontario Superior Court ruled that the determination of death was made in accordance with "accepted medical practice," so McKitty had no constitutional right to the freedom of religion, but a Court of Appeal judge overruled this decision on the grounds that there was no consideration of whether the determination of BD/DNC was constitutional. However, she had a circulatory-respiratory arrest before completion of the appeal process and no decision was rendered because the dispute was moot.

(continued on next page)

Table 3 (continued)	
RL (Ireland, United Kingdom)[35] 2022	RL was a 21-year-old man who had hypoxic-ischemic brain injury after anaphylaxis. He was declared brain dead/dead by neurologic criteria, but his parents objected and tried to facilitate transfer to a private clinic in another country under the care of a clinician who did not accept the concept of BD/DNC. The High Court ruled that death was appropriately determined and the clinician offering to allow RL to be transferred to their clinic added to his parents' grief by providing them unrealistic and false hope. The High Court gave the hospital permission to discontinue organ support.

consent to perform an evaluation for the determination of BD/DNC.[40,41] First, clinicians are obliged to make the important and fundamental distinction between life and death. Second, because performing an evaluation to determine death by circulatory-respiratory criteria does not require consent, it would be inconsistent to require consent before performing an evaluation for determination of BD/DNC. Third, a determination of death should not be negotiable. Finally, consideration of distributive justice and the scarcity of resources, such as critical care beds, argues against requesting consent to determine death.

For all of these reasons, the AAN and the World Brain Death Project both note that consent is not required to determine BD/DNC, and no state legally requires consent to perform this evaluation.[19,20,41] However, both the AAN and World Brain Death Project advise family notification of the intent to perform a BD/DNC evaluation.[19,20] This requirement is also explicitly noted in both the Nevada statute and New York guidelines on determination of death.[42,43]

SHOULD ORGAN SUPPORT BE CONTINUED UNTIL CIRCULATORY-RESPIRATORY ARREST IF A FAMILY OBJECTS TO BRAIN DEATH/DEATH BY NEUROLOGIC CRITERIA?

Although there are ethical arguments in both support of and opposition to accommodation of objections to BD/DNC (**Table 4**), most clinicians involved in the determination of BD/DNC do not think organ support should be continued after determination of BD/DNC until circulatory-respiratory arrest.[23,34,44] A survey of neurologists from the United States found that only 16% of respondents thought that every state should legally allow accommodation of objections to BD/DNC.[34]

At present, although no states require consent to evaluate for BD/DNC, four states accommodate objections to BD/DNC: California and New York require "reasonable" efforts to accommodate religious/cultural/moral objections to BD/DNC[42,45]; Illinois requires a patient's religious beliefs to be "taken into account" when determining time of death[46]; and in New Jersey, death can only be declared by circulatory-respiratory criteria if a patient has a religious objection to BD/DNC.[47]

The AAN and the World Brain Death Project do not endorse continuation of organ support until circulatory-respiratory arrest after BD/DNC has been established even if a family objects to BD/DNC.[19,20] The AAN supports "requests for limited accommodation based on reasonable and sincere social, moral, cultural, and religious considerations" but "recognizes that when attempts to reconcile disputes pertaining to indefinite accommodation fail, unilateral withdrawal of organ-sustaining technology (other than in pregnant women) over the objection of loved ones is acceptable, when supported by law and institutional policy, and represents a measure of last resort."[19] Similarly, the World Brain Death Project notes accommodation of objections

Table 4
Ethical principles that support/refute accommodation of objections to death/death by neurologic criteria

Ethical Principle	Perspective	Application of Ethical Principles to Management of Objections to the Use of Neurologic Criteria to Declare Death	
		Support for Accommodation	Opposition to Accommodation
Beneficence	Patient	• Continuation of organ support at the request of the LAR, who should be considered an extension of the patient, can be considered support of the patient's freedom of religion, dignity, and autonomy	
	LAR	• Continuation of organ support can allow the LAR to come to terms with the patient's death	
	Health-care professionals	• Continuation of organ support at the request of the LAR fulfills the obligation of health-care professionals to act in ways that benefit their patients and by extension LARs of patients who lack capacity	
	Society	• Continuation of organ support at the request of the LAR can be considered support of the societal principles of freedom of religion and respect for autonomy	
Nonmaleficence	Patient	• Discontinuation of organ support despite the objection of the LAR, who should be considered an extension of the patient, can be considered a violation of the patient's dignity and autonomy	• Continuation of organ support after death could be considered disrespectful to the patient if the LAR is not aware of/representing their true beliefs and wishes • Continuation of organ support after death can be considered a violation of the patient's dignity if the LAR is not aware of/representing their true beliefs and wishes
	LAR	• Discontinuation of organ support despite the objection of the LAR could lead to moral and psychological distress for the LAR, who should be considered an extension of the patient	• Continuation of organ support after death may cause harm by preventing closure and increasing the risk for complicated grief for the LAR
	Health-care professionals	• Discontinuation of organ support despite the objection of the LAR could lead to moral and psychological distress for health-care professionals • Discontinuation of organ support despite the objection of the LAR may cause health-care professionals to be concerned they are violating the societal principles of freedom of religion and respect for autonomy	• Continuation of organ support after death may lead to moral distress for health-care professionals • Continuation of organ support after death may cause health-care professionals to be concerned they are being disrespectful to the patient • Continuation of organ support after death may cause health-care professionals to be concerned they are violating the patient's dignity

(continued on next page)

Table 4
(continued)

		Application of Ethical Principles to Management of Objections to the Use of Neurologic Criteria to Declare Death	
Ethical Principle	Perspective	Support for Accommodation	Opposition to Accommodation
	Society	• Discontinuation of organ support despite the objection of the LAR can be considered a harmful violation of the societal principles of freedom of religion and respect for autonomy	• Continuation of organ support after death may cause health-care professionals to be concerned they are violating the societal principles of equity and universality • Continuation of organ support after death can be considered a harmful violation of the societal principles of equity and universality
Respect for autonomy	Patient LAR Health-care professionals Society	• Respect for patient autonomy • Freedom of religion • Respect for LAR autonomy • Freedom of religion • Freedom of religion	• Respect for the autonomy of health-care professionals
Justice	Patient LAR Health-care professionals Society	• Organ support can be continued after death by neurologic criteria if a patient is pregnant or organ donation is planned, so it should also be continued if there is an objection to the use of neurologic criteria to declare death	• Principles of equity and universality argue against a negotiated standard for what happens after death by neurologic criteria since objections to death by cardiopulmonary criteria are not accepted • Health-care resources (including an intensive care unit bed, medical equipment, medications and health-care professionals' time) are intended for patients who are alive • Insurance company funds are intended for patients who are alive

Abbreviation: LAR, legally-authorized representation.

From Lewis A. Should the Revised Uniform Determination of Death Act Address Objections to the Use of Neurologic Criteria to Declare Death?. Neurocrit Care. 2022;37(2):377-385; with permission.

to BD/DNC for a finite period of time is reasonable, assuming that the specific time frame for doing so is brief and uniform (<48 hours).[20]

THE FUTURE OF MANAGEMENT OF OBJECTIONS TO BRAIN DEATH/DEATH BY NEUROLOGIC CRITERIA

Clinicians involved in determining BD/DNC often feel uncomfortable handling objections to BD/DNC and think that something needs to be done to make these objections easier to handle.[23,34] Clear, universal legal guidance to manage objections to BD/DNC would improve management of objections to BD/DNC for patients, families, the health-care team, hospitals, and society and may help minimize friction and mistrust between clinicians and families.

In light of the escalating frequency of objections to BD/DNC, discussions are underway about potential revisions to the UDDA. It is unclear whether a revised UDDA would include guidance on managing objections to BD/DNC and what that guidance would be.[44] However, some potential approaches include (1) indefinite continuation of organ support until declaration of death by circulatory-respiratory criteria, (2) a brief period of accommodation, (3) consideration of religious beliefs when determining time of death, or (4) discontinuation of organ support despite objections to BD/DNC.[48]

Until there is further legal guidance about management of objections to BD/DNC, clinicians can strive to mitigate controversy about BD/DNC via empathetic, culturally sensitive discussions about BD/DNC that incorporate palliative care specialists, chaplain services, and social work to support families and mitigate escalation to the courts. Additionally, hospitals should create policies that address the management of objections to BD/DNC to facilitate internal practice consistency.

SUMMARY

Medicolegal acceptance of BD/DNC has grown since the 1960s, but the concept continues to face ethical and legal challenges. Objections to BD/DNC are typically grounded in religious beliefs. Unfortunately, neither hospitals nor state laws provide adequate standardized guidance about how best to address objections to BD/DNC. Therefore, the management of objections to BD/DNC varies. Patients, families, health-care teams, hospitals, and society would all benefit from uniform medicolegal guidance about the management of objections to BD/DNC across states (and around the world).

CLINICS CARE POINTS

- Educate families of patients with catastrophic brain injury about the risk for progression to BD/DNC
- Inform families of the intent to perform an evaluation to determine BD/DNC
- Incorporate pastoral care, social work, and palliative care in discussions about BD/DNC to provide family support
- Develop a hospital protocol to manage objections to BD/DNC

DISCLOSURES

A. Lewis is an observer on the Uniform Law Commission Drafting Committee on Updating the Uniform Determination of Death and received a stipend for editing "Death Determination by Neurologic Criteria: Areas of Controversy and Consensus."

REFERENCES

1. Beck CS, Pritchard WH, Feil HS. Ventricular fibrillation of long duration abolished by electric shock. J Am Med Assoc 1947;135(15):985–6.
2. Diagnosis and Treatment of the Acute Phase of Poliomyelitis and its Complications. Postgrad Med J 1955;31(358). https://doi.org/10.1136/pgmj.31.358.420-b.
3. Mollaret P, Goulon M. The depassed coma (preliminary memoir). Rev Neurol (Paris) 1959;101:3–15.
4. Gilder SSB. Twenty-second World Medical Assembly. Br Med J 1968;3(5616): 493–4.
5. Beecher HK. A Definition of Irreversible Coma: Report of the Ad Hoc Committee of the Harvard Medical School to Examine the Definition of Brain Death. JAMA 1968;205(6):337–40.
6. Wijdicks EFM. How Harvard Defined Irreversible Coma. Neurocrit Care 2018; 29(1):136–41.
7. Lewis A, Scheyer O. Legal Objections to Use of Neurologic Criteria to Declare Death in the United States: 1968 to 2017. Chest 2019;155(6):1234–45.
8. Wigodsky HS. Deciding to Forego Life-Sustaining Treatment: A Report on the Ethical, Medical, and Legal Issues in Treatment Decisions. JAMA, J Am Med Assoc 1984;251(14):1903–4.
9. Diagnosis of brain death. Statement issued by the honorary secretary of the Conference of Medical Royal Colleges and their Faculties in the United Kingdom on 11 October 1976. Br Med J 1976;2(6045):1187–8.
10. Wijdicks EFM. The transatlantic divide over brain death determination and the debate. Brain 2012;135(4):1321–31.
11. President's Commission for the Study of Ethical Problems in Medicine and Biomedical and Behavioral Research Appointment of the Membership and Nomination of the Chairman. | The American Presidency Project. Available at: https://www.presidency.ucsb.edu/documents/presidents-commission-for-the-study-ethical-problems-medicine-and-biomedical-and-1. Accessed January 21, 2023.
12. Defining Death: Medical, Legal and Ethical Issues in the Determination of Death. Washington D.C.; 1981.
13. Lewis A, Cahn-Fuller K, Caplan A. Shouldn't dead be dead?: The search for a uniform definition of death. J Law Med Ethics 2017;45(1):112–28.
14. Report of special Task Force. Guidelines for the determination of brain death in children. American Academy of Pediatrics Task Force on Brain Death in Children. Pediatrics 1987;80(2):298–300.
15. Nakagawa TA, Ashwal S, Mathur M, et al. Guidelines for the determination of brain death in infants and children: An update of the 1987 Task Force recommendations. Crit Care Med 2011;39(9):2139–55.
16. Wijdicks EFM. Determining brain death in adults. Neurology 1995;45(5):1003–11.
17. Wijdicks EFM, Varelas PN, Gronseth GS, et al. Evidence-based guideline update: Determining brain death in adults. Neurology 2010;74(23):1911–8.
18. American Academy of Neurology: Neurology Resources | AAN. Available at: https://www.aan.com/. Accessed January 25, 2023.
19. Russell JA, Epstein LG, Greer DM, et al. Brain death, the determination of brain death, and member guidance for brain death accommodation requests: AAN position statement. Neurology 2019;92(5):228–32.
20. Greer DM, Shemie SD, Lewis A, et al. Determination of Brain Death/Death by Neurologic Criteria: The World Brain Death Project. JAMA, J Am Med Assoc 2020;324(11):1078–97.

21. Lewis A, Bakkar A, Kreiger-Benson E, et al. Determination of death by neurologic criteria around the world. Neurology 2020;95(3):E299–309.

22. Lewis A, Lord AS, Czeisler BM, et al. Public education and misinformation on brain death in mainstream media. Clin Transplant 2016;30(9):1082–9.

23. Lewis A, Adams N, Chopra A, et al. Organ Support after Death by Neurologic Criteria in Pediatric Patients. Crit Care Med 2017;45(9):E916–24.

24. Lewis A, Caplan A. Brain death in the media. Transplantation 2016;100(5):E24.

25. Daoust A, Racine E. Depictions of "brain death" in the media: medical and ethical implications. J Med Ethics 2014;40(4):253–9.

26. Lewis A, Weaver J, Caplan A. Portrayal of Brain Death in Film and Television. Am J Transplant 2017;17(3):761–9.

27. Zheng K, Sutherland S, Hornby L, et al. Public Understandings of the Definition and Determination of Death: A Scoping Review. Transplant Direct 2022;8(5): E1300.

28. Lewis A, Varelas P, Greer D. Prolonging Support After Brain Death: When Families Ask for More. Neurocrit Care 2016;24(3):481–7.

29. van Beinum A, Healey A, Chandler J, et al. Requests for somatic support after neurologic death determination: Canadian physician experiences. Can J Anaesth 2021;68(3):293.

30. To the 18th International Congress of the Transplantation Society (2000) | John Paul II. Available at: https://www.vatican.va/content/john-paul-ii/en/speeches/2000/jul-sep/documents/hf_jp-ii_spe_20000829_transplants.html. Accessed January 22, 2023.

31. Lewis A, Kitamura E. The Intersection of Neurology and Religion: A Survey of Hospital Chaplains on Death by Neurologic Criteria. Neurocrit Care 2021;35(2): 322–34.

32. Lewis A. A Survey of Multidenominational Rabbis on Death by Neurologic Criteria. Neurocrit Care 2019;31(2):411–8.

33. Lewis A, Kitamura E, Padela AI. Allied Muslim Healthcare Professional Perspectives on Death by Neurologic Criteria. Neurocrit Care 2020;33(2):347–57.

34. Lewis A, Adams N, Varelas P, et al. Organ support after death by neurologic criteria: Results of a survey of US neurologists. Neurology 2016;87(8):827–34.

35. Lewis A. An Overview of Ethical Issues Raised by Medicolegal Challenges to Death by Neurologic Criteria in the United Kingdom and a Comparison to Management of These Challenges in the USA. Am J Bioeth 2023;1–18.

36. Lewis A, Greer D. Medicolegal Complications of Apnoea Testing for Determination of Brain Death. J bioeth Inq 2018;15(3):417–28.

37. Shewmon DA. POINT: Whether Informed Consent Should Be Obtained for Apnea Testing in the Determination of Death by Neurologic Criteria? Yes. Chest 2022; 161(5):1143–5.

38. Muramoto O. Is informed consent required for the diagnosis of brain death regardless of consent for organ donation? J Med Ethics 2021;47(12):E5.

39. Truog RD, Tasker RC. COUNTERPOINT: Should Informed Consent Be Required for Apnea Testing in Patients With Suspected Brain Death? Yes. Chest 2017; 152(4):702–4.

40. Pope TM. COUNTERPOINT: Whether Informed Consent Should Be Obtained for Apnea Testing in the Determination of Death by Neurologic Criteria? No. Chest 2022;161(5):1145–7.

41.. Pope TM. Is consent required for clinicians to make a determination of death by neurologic criteria?. In: Lewis A, Bernat JL, editors. *Death determination by neurologic criteria: areas of controversy and consensus.* Switzerland: Springer Nature; 2023. p. 287–303.

42. Guidelines for Determining Brain Death. Available at: https://www.health.ny.gov/professionals/hospital_administrator/letters/2011/brain_death_guidelines.htm. Accessed January 25, 2023.

43. AB424 Overview. Accessed January 25, 2023. Available at: https://www.leg.state.nv.us/App/NELIS/REL/79th2017/Bill/5570/Overview.

44. Lewis A. Should the Revised Uniform Determination of Death Act Address Objections to the Use of Neurologic Criteria to Declare Death? Neurocrit Care 2022; 37(2):377–85.

45. AB 2565 Assembly Bill. Accessed January 25, 2023. Available at: http://www.leginfo.ca.gov/pub/07-08/bill/asm/ab_2551-2600/ab_2565_bill_20080927_chaptered.html.

46. 210 ILCS 85/Hospital Licensing Act. Accessed January 25, 2023. Available at: https://www.ilga.gov/legislation/ilcs/ilcs3.asp?ActID=1234&ChapterID=21.

47. (New Jersey) Declaration of Death Act (NJDDA) - 01/18/2013 — New Jersey Law Revision Commission. Accessed January 25, 2023. Available at: https://www.njlrc.org/projects/2019/6/5/new-jersey-adult-guardianship-and-protective-proceedings-jurisdiction-act-z35cb-bear6-bnshg.

48. Lewis A. The Uniform Determination of Death Act is Being Revised. Neurocrit Care 2022;36(2):335–8.

49. Bresnahan MJ, Mahler K. Ethical debate over organ donation in the context of brain death. Bioethics 2010;24(2):54–60.

50. Son RG, Setta SM. Frequency of use of the religious exemption in New Jersey cases of determination of brain death. BMC Med Ethics 2018;19(1):76.

51. Mizuno T, Slingsby BT. Eye on religion: Considering the influence of Buddhist and Shinto thought on contemporary Japanese bioethics. South Med J 2007;100(1): 115–7.

52. Ostertag C, Karches K. Brain Death and the Formation of Moral Conscience. Linacre Q 2019;86(4). https://doi.org/10.1177/0024363919872622.

53. Sgreccia E. Vegetative state and brain death: Philosophical and ethical issues from a personalistic view. NeuroRehabilitation 2004;19(4):361–6.

54. Miller AC. Opinions on the Legitimacy of Death Declaration by Neurological Criteria from the Perspective of 3 Abrahamic Faiths. Medeni Med J 2019;34(3): 305–13.

55.. Campbell C. Christian perspectives on death by neurologic criteria. In: Lewis A, Bernat JL, editors. *Death determination by neurologic criteria: areas of controversy and consensus.* Switzerland: Springer Nature; 2023. p. 341–56.

56. Hinduism, Brain Death, Organ Transplantation | HuffPost Religion. Accessed January 22, 2023. Available at: https://www.huffpost.com/entry/hinduism-brain-death-orga_b_12198832.

57. Alhawari Y, Verhoff MA, Parzeller M. Brain death, organ transplantation and autopsy from the point of view of world religions: Part 2: Hinduism, Buddhism, Shintoism, Taoism, discussion, conclusion. Rechtsmedizin 2018;28(4):272–9.

58. Setta SM, Shemie SD. An explanation and analysis of how world religions formulate their ethical decisions on withdrawing treatment and determining death. Philos Ethics Humanit Med 2015;10(1). https://doi.org/10.1186/s13010-015-0025-x.

59. Miller AC, Ziad-Miller A, Elamin EM. Brain death and Islam: The interface of religion, culture, history, law, and modern medicine. Chest 2014;146(4):1071–5.

60.. Padela AI, Rahid R. Islamic perspectives on death by neurologic criteria. In: Lewis A, Bernat JL, editors. *Death determination by neurologic criteria: areas of controversy and consensus*. Switzerland: Springer Nature; 2023. p. 357–79.

61. Weiss DW. Organ transplantation, medical ethics, and Jewish law. Transplant Proc 1988;20(1 Suppl 1):1071–5.

62. Rappaport ZH, Rappaport IT. Brain death and organ transplantation: concepts and principles in Judaism. Adv Exp Med Biol 2004;550:133–7. https://doi.org/10.1007/978-0-306-48526-8_10.

63. Rappaport ZH, Rappaport IT. Principles and concepts of brain death and organ donation: The Jewish perspective. Acta Neurochir Suppl 1999;1999(SUPPL. 74):61–3.

64.. Shabtai D. Jewish perspectives on death by neurologic criteria. In: Lewis A, Bernat JL, editors. *Death determination by neurologic criteria: areas of controversy and consensus*. Switzerland: Springer Nature; 2023. p. 381–93.

65. Feldman EA. Defining death: Organ transplants, tradition and technology in Japan. Soc Sci Med 1988;27(4):339–43.

66.. Mathis BJ, Terunuma Y, Hiramatsu Y. Cultural considerations in the declaration of death by neurologic criteria in Asia. In: Lewis A, Bernat JL, editors. *Death determination by neurologic criteria: areas of controversy and consensus*. Switzerland: Springer Nature; 2023. p. 405–26.

67. Lewis A. Reconciling the Case of Jahi McMath. Neurocrit Care 2018;29(1):20–2.

68. Aviv R. What does it mean to Die? | the new Yorker. The New Yorker; 2018.

69. Yanke G, Rady MY, Verheijde JL. In re guardianship of Hailu: The Nevada Supreme Court casts doubt on the standard for brain death diagnosis. Med Sci Law 2017;57(2):100–2.

70. Lewis A, Greer D. Current controversies in brain death determination. Nat Rev Neurol 2017;13(8):505–9.

71.. Chandler JA. Legal responses to religious and other objections to declaration of death by neurologic criteria. In: Lewis A, Bernat JL, editors. *Death determination by neurologic criteria: areas of controversy and consensus*. Switzerland: Springer Nature; 2023. p. 305–20.

Medical Malpractice and the Neurologist: An Introduction

James C. Johnston, MD, JD[a,b],*, Thomas P. Sartwelle, BBA, LLB[c]

KEYWORDS

- Medical malpractice • Neurologic malpractice • Expert witness • Negligence
- Standard of care

KEY POINTS

- A malpractice claim requires the injured patient to prove four elements by a preponderance of evidence: the physician owed a duty to conform to a recognized standard of care and breached that duty, leading to the proximate cause of injury and resulting in legally cognizable damages.
- The standard of care may be conflated with practice guidelines which necessitates careful documentation for any deviation from guideline recommendations.
- There are numerous claims beyond negligence that may be filed simultaneously with a malpractice suit.
- Neurology is a high-risk specialty based on the absolute number of paid claims, payment ratio, average indemnity payment, and defense costs for closed claims and paid claims.
- Expert witness practices engender unique risks that require particular attention.

MALPRACTICE LIABILITY

Defining Malpractice

The torts most applicable to the medical profession are negligence (professional as opposed to ordinary or gross) and the intentional torts involving trespass to the person (eg, battery, assault, false imprisonment, intentional infliction of emotional distress). Negligence is the name of a broad omnibus tort cause of action as well as the term ascribed to conduct falling below the standard established by law to protect others against unreasonable risks of harm.

Author contributions: The authors contributed equally to the research, development, writing, review, and approval of the content.

Declaration of conflicting interests: The authors declared no potential conflicts of interest with respect to the research, authorship, and publication of this article.

Funding: The authors received no financial support for the research, authorship, and publication of this article.

a GlobalNeurology®, 52917B Farnham Street, Auckland 1052, New Zealand; b GlobalNeurology®, 5290 Medical Drive, San Antonio, TX 78229, USA; c Hicks Davis Wynn, PC, 3555 Timmons Lane, Suite 1000, Houston, TX 77027, USA

* Corresponding author. 52917B Farnham Street, Auckland 1052, New Zealand; 5290 Medical Drive, San Antonio, TX 78229.

E-mail address: johnston@GlobalNeurology.com

Neurol Clin 41 (2023) 485–491

https://doi.org/10.1016/j.ncl.2023.05.001

0733-8619/23/© 2023 Elsevier Inc. All rights reserved.

neurologic.theclinics.com

Medical negligence refers to professional negligence by a health care provider—a physician fails to exercise the degree of care and skill ordinarily used by the medical profession under the same or similar circumstances and conditions.

A *prima facie* medical negligence or malpractice claim mandates that the injured patient prove four elements by a preponderance of evidence.

1. The physician owing a duty to conform to a recognized standard of professional care;
2. Breached that duty;
3. Which was the proximate cause of an injury;
4. Resulting in legally cognizable damages.

There are various legal issues surrounding each element—judicially devised restrictions to limit the boundaries of liability.

For example, in medical malpractice, the duty owed by a defendant physician arises from the physician–patient relationship; alleged negligence must occur within the course of that relationship. Regarding the first element, owing a duty, does a telephone conversation with a prospective patient create a relationship? Will being on call impose the requisite duty? Reading an electroencephalogram? What about the consulting neurologist discussing a case with the treating physician? And once a relationship is established, what does the duty entail? How does a physician end the duty?

The second element, breach of duty, is perhaps the most controversial and discussed below under standard of care.

Causation, the third element, is a complex query involving two factual issues: First, was the physician's alleged negligence a proximate cause of the injury, or was there an intervening cause? Second, were the injuries a foreseeable result of the physician's substandard care? The law of causation varies widely among jurisdictions; *Daubert*[a] allows courts broad discretion in deciding what scientific evidence is admissible.

The fourth element requires actual damages, or there is no cause of action. The breach of a professional duty causing nominal damages, speculative harm, or possible future harm does not constitute a malpractice action.

The statutes of limitations vary by state but generally include two periods—the deadline to file a claim, which starts when the malpractice occurred; and most jurisdictions have an exception so that the time limit does not start until the patient discovers or reasonably should have discovered the malpractice.

These queries and related legal issues are beyond the ambit of this brief introduction.[1] The clinician should simply recognize that each element of a negligence claim may raise a host of legal arguments.

STANDARD OF CARE

Most medical malpractice litigation focuses on whether the physician breached or departed from the standard of care, an argument that may center on practice

---

[a] The Daubert standard is the standard used by a trial judge to assess whether an expert witness's scientific testimony is based on scientifically valid reasoning which can properly be applied to the facts at issue. This standard comes from the Supreme Court case Daubert v Merrell Dow Pharmaceuticals Inc, 509 US 579 (1993). Under the Daubert standard, the factors that may be considered in determining whether the methodology is valid are (1) whether the theory or technique in question can be and has been tested; (2) whether it has been subjected to peer review and publication; (3) its known or potential error rate; (4) the existence and maintenance of standards controlling its operation; and (5) whether it has attracted widespread acceptance within a relevant scientific community. https://www.law.cornell.edu/wex/daubert_standard#:~:text=The%20Daubert%20standard%20is%20the,to%20the%20facts%20at%20issue. Accessed April 23, 2023.

parameters or evidence-based guidelines. These guidelines may be admissible if qualified as authoritative, thereby avoiding hearsay limitations. Some courts have adopted a more liberal approach by admitting clinical guidelines as demonstrative aids, noting that such an extrajudicial statement "would only be classic hearsay if it was offered to prove the truth of the matter asserted therein."[2] This is a particular concern for clinicians as the medical profession including the American Academy of Neurology (AAN) publishes an ever-increasing number of evidence-based guides for the management of specific diseases. The National Guideline Clearinghouse closed on 18 July 2018, but a current search of the Agency for Healthcare Research and Quality using the term "neurology guidelines" uncovers several hundred articles of varying quality, a search of the AAN Web site lists 80 neurology-specific guidelines which were developed, reviewed, or revised within the preceding 5 years, and the European Academy of Neurology has 161 active guidelines.[3] These guidelines are not inflexible and should be viewed as an accepted course of treatment rather than the final arbiter of a standard of care. Many, if not all, have a generic disclaimer to that effect. However, a negligence claim alleging harm because of transgression from a guideline represents a strong argument. Neurologists should carefully document any treatment decisions that deviate from practice guidelines.

MALPRACTICE BEYOND NEGLIGENCE

Medical malpractice claims most commonly allege negligence but may be brought simultaneously under several legal theories including wrongful death; lack of informed consent; battery and assault; loss of chance; abandonment; negligent referral; breach of contract; breach of privacy or confidentiality; negligent infliction of emotional distress; failure to warn; defamation; fraud and misrepresentation; failure to report; products liability for drugs or devices; loss of consortium; and vicarious liability.

These claims may be quite powerful and, for the plaintiff, more effective than an allegation of negligence. For example, battery may be claimed when a procedure is performed differently than agreed on during the informed consent process or when the patient refused or withdrew consent. Medical battery, unlike negligence, does not require proof of a duty or breach of duty. The plaintiff does not have to incur any physical injury. Expert testimony is not required to award damages. Moreover, it is an intentional tort, thereby allowing punitive damages in addition to damages for mental anguish. Malpractice caps on damages do not apply to battery. In another example, breach of contract may be claimed because it generally has a longer statute of limitations than negligence and expert witness testimony is not necessary for the case to go to the jury.

General Remarks on Malpractice

The provision of medical care meeting or even exceeding the prevailing standard may not shield the neurologist from a lawsuit. A solid physician–patient relationship, valid consent, and proper medical record documentation are essential for successful risk management and malpractice defense. The root of a malpractice claim is injury or perceived injury; however, most suits are triggered by a breakdown in the physician–patient relationship due to poor communication. A thorough understanding of this relationship improves communication, thereby meeting patients' expectations, significantly reducing the risk of suit. Informed consent issues are a frequent source of claims wholly unrelated to negligence lawsuits, and the legal theories are detailed in the literature. Poor documentation remains the leading factor in the forced settlement of most malpractice claims. The literature is replete with recommendations for ensuring that records are clear, accurate, complete, legible, and timely without alter-ations or other evidence of spoliation. It would be redundant to reiterate good record-keeping principles, but one legal maxim must be emphasized: *If it is not in the record, it never happened.*

Current trends in malpractice

The overall medical malpractice claims frequency (number of claims filed) in the United States is at a historic low dropping 27% in the decade up to 2016 before slowing, but the expenses and indemnity payments increased, especially payments exceeding 1 million dollars.[4–6] However, the trend varies by specialty and there is a paradoxically adverse impact on neurology. In a recent survey, 62% of neurologists and neurosur-geons have been named in at least one malpractice suit.[7] The cumulative data from an insurance consortium review of closed neurology claim since 1988 combined with data from the 2019 survey paints a disconcerting picture.[8]

- The absolute number of paid neurology claims has remained steady over the past decade (without a significant change in number of closed claims).
- The payment ratio (percentage of paid claims to claims closed) remains high (24.52%), exceeding every preceding 5-year interval average for the past 25 years.
- Neurology had the highest average indemnity payment through 2008 and then decreased slightly to $416,835, exceeding all specialties except neurosurgery ($22,311 higher).
- Among cases that resulted in a settlement or verdict in favor of the plaintiff, one-third reached $500,000, 27% at 1 million, and 19% exceeded 2 million.
- Neurology claims are costly to defend—average expenses paid for closed claims and paid claims increasing significantly over the recent years.

Neurology: a high risk specialty?

There are several unique factors inherent to the specialty that may explain these para-doxic findings, which remain at odds with the general malpractice trends. First, the un-precedented growth of sophisticated neurodiagnostic tests, the proliferation of neuropharmacological agents, and the advent of more invasive procedures raise the standard of care, increasing the level of accountability and hence likelihood of suit. Second, neurologists confront a diverse array of legal issues beyond the scope of traditional practice involving, among others, brain death, genetic testing, compe-tency issues, neurotoxic insults, and evaluation of the neurologically impaired child. These varied conditions—governed by expanding legal doctrines, evolving regulatory control, and political whims—expose the neurologist to novel claims. Third, neurologic liability extends beyond the physician–patient relationship to a host of third parties. For example, there is tort liability for negligence to a patient that also injures a fetus, child, or spouse. In addition to the duty to warn of imminently dangerous patients, there is now a duty to warn third parties of communicable diseases. Neurologists have a duty to warn patients of medical conditions that may impair driving (epilepsy, sleep disorders, movement disorders, and stroke); they may also be required to warn others directly, either by statute or an imposed tort duty to warn of foreseeable harm. The result is an ever-expanding pool of potential claimants. Fourth, the very nature of neurologic disease or injury spells a grave outcome for many patients, and this is re-flected in the high-indemnity payments.

The confluence of medical advancements, diverse legal trends, and sociopolitical movements has transformed neurology from a low-risk specialty to one plagued by high-indemnity claims, with a high payment ratio that are costly to defend.

Neurologic claims related to the pandemic

The severe acute respiratory syndrome coronavirus 2 (SARS-CoV-2) pandemic unleashed from Wuhan, China in 2019 rapidly seeded the entire world and dramatically changed the practice of medicine from temporary bans on elective procedures to the rise of telemedicine. There may be novel claims related to the diagnosis and treatment of COVID-19 including vaccine-related neurologic injuries, although there are hurdles such as the Coronavirus Aid, Relief, and Economic Security Act. Allegations of failure to protect patients from the virus may arise. There are myriad potential claims from the use of telemedicine. At this point in time, it is too early to determine the impact that this pandemic may have on malpractice claims.

NON-MALPRACTICE LIABILITY

Neurologists must be cognizant of the far-reaching laws and regulations affecting their practice, raising the specter of adverse licensing sanctions, civil penalties, and criminal prosecution. This non-malpractice liability penumbra generically includes credentialing disputes (eg, professional licensure, hospital privileges, professional organization membership), reimbursement issues (eg, fee disputes, program exclusion, denial of managed care contracts), and myriad ad personam, economic, and regulatory crimes. The relevant legal principles governing these diverse areas are substantially different among various jurisdictions and thus beyond the scope of this article.

FORENSIC NEUROLOGY LIABILITY: THE EXPERT WITNESS

Neurologists performing medical record reviews, independent medical examinations, and expert witness services engender unique risks.[9] Some jurisdictions may allow malpractice claims for third party examinations; others assign a limited physician–patient relationship, opening the door for ordinary negligence claims.

There are numerous anecdotal reports of neurologists advancing specious complaints,[10] an ongoing problem described four decades ago with a review that documented neurologists providing improper expert testimony in 37% of cases.[11] It is "alarmingly common for accomplished neurologists to hire themselves out for [one-sided testimony]."[12] These partisan experts have flourished behind the common law expert witness immunity doctrine and lack of professional oversight. Today, there is a trend toward accountability with increased expert witness liability. Friendly expert lawsuits (retaining party sues the expert) are increasing. The traditional immunity is not absolute, and many states ruling on this issue have carved out exceptions to hold the expert liable for professional negligence.[13] One state Supreme Court explained that an "absence of immunity will protect the litigant from the negligence of an incompetent professional."[14] In addition, courts have upheld suits against opposing and independent experts. Some jurisdictions continue to favor immunity for testimony but that does not necessarily extend to nontestimonial expert activity (eg, discovery of facts, literature search). Nor does it protect the expert from criminal prosecution for improper testimony or misrepresentation of a degree or license. The expert neurologist may also be liable for defamatory communications and face administrative, civil, or criminal charges for negligent or intentional spoliation of evidence.

Expert testimony and related activities are subject to increasing scrutiny by state licensing boards and professional organizations. The American Medical Association considers testimony to be the practice of medicine and subject to peer review and supports state licensing boards in disciplining physicians who provide fraudulent testimony or false credentials. Some boards have expanded the definition of medical practice to include testimony, allowing disciplinary action if warranted. The AANs Code of Professional Conduct explicitly states that expert witness qualifications and testimony must comport with the *AAN Qualifications and Guidelines for the Physician Expert Witness*.[15,16] The AAN Disciplinary Action Policy outlines a formal disciplinary procedure for errant neurologists with potential sanctions ranging from censure to expulsion.[17,18] AAN disciplinary actions may trigger the American Board of Psychiatry and Neurology to revoke certification.[19] The Seventh Circuit Court of Appeals validated these forms of discipline, stating in dicta that the American Academy of Neurologic Surgeons had a duty to discipline a neurosurgeon for irresponsible testimony.[20]

This complex evolving area of law creates a more perilous liability climate for the expert witness. The standard of care varies with the particular facts of each case, but salient guidelines generally applicable in all jurisdictions include the following: fulfill the relevant qualifications before accepting a case; review all relevant medical information; review the standard of care for the time of occurrence; perform adequate discovery of facts; review and understand the relevant literature; properly assemble and present the case; avoid losing or destroying any evidence; provide accurate, impartial, and truthful testimony; avoid conflicts of interest; do not discuss the case outside the course of litigation; and ensure compensation is reasonable, not contingent on outcome. It is important to remember that deposition and trial testimony generally constitutes a permanent public record, which may be readily accessed from various national repositories.[21]

Portions of the text are updated from James C. Johnston, Neurologic malpractice and non-malpractice liability, Neurol Clin 2010; 28(2):441-458, with permission.

REFERENCES

1. Louisell DW, Williams H. Medical Malpractice. LexisNexis Matthew Bender Elite Products. In: Beran R, editor. Legal and forensic medicine. Berlin, Germany: springer-Verlag publishing, 2013. Wecht CH, ed. Preparing and Winning medical negligence cases. New York: Juris Publishing; 2022. p. 2009.
2. Hinlicky v. Dreyfuss (2006) 848 N.E.2d 1285 (carotid endarterectomy guideline serves as a "demonstrative aid for the jury in understanding the process" that defendant followed in caring for patient).
3. Available at: https://search.ahrq.gov/. Accessed January 28, 2023; www.aan.com. Accessed January 28, 2023; https://www.ean.org/research/ean-guidelines/guideline-reference-center. Accessed January 28, 2023.
4. Aon/ASHRM Hospital and Physician Professional Liability. Benchmark Analysis, September 2022. Available at: https://www.candello.com/Solutions/Data. Accessed December 4, 2022.
5. 2018 Benchmarking report. Medical malpractice in America. See, Baker T. The medical malpractice Myth. Chicago (Il)l: Univ of Chicago Press; 2005.
6. Available at: https://www.npdb.hrsa.gov/analysistool/. Accessed January 6, 2023.
7. Martin KL. Medscape Neurologist Malpractice Report 2019. Available at: https://www.medscape.com/slideshow/2019-malpractice-report-neuro-6012448. Accessed December 12, 2022.
8. Physicians Insurers Association of America. Risk management review (neurology). Rockville, MD: PIAA 2013. See also Aon/ASHMR Hospital and Physician Liability Benchmark Analysis 2021.
9. Johnston JC, Sartwelle TP. The expert witness in medical malpractice litigation: through the looking glass. J Child Neurol 2013;28(4):484–501.

10. Sartwelle TP, Johnston JC. Continuous electronic fetal monitoring during labor: a critique and a reply to contemporary proponents. Surg J 2018;4:e23–8.
11. Id Safran A, Skydell B, Ropper S. Expert witness testimony in neurology: Massachusetts experience 1980-1990. Neurol Chronicle 1992;44:2477–84.
12. Supra note 97. Holtz S. The neurologist as an expert witness. AAN Education Program Syllabus 7DS.003 (2002).
13. Butz v. Economou, 438 U.S. 478 (1978). See also Restatement (Second) of Torts §588 (limiting immunity to statements that have "some relation to the proceeding").
14. Marrogi v. Howard, 805 So.2d 1118 (La. 2002) (holding there was no immunity for either pretrial work or trial testimony).
15. Russell JA, Hutchins JC, Epstein LG, on behalf of the AAN Ethics, Law, and Humanities Committee. American Academy of Neurology Code of Professional Conduct. Neurology 2021;97(10):489–95.
16. American Academy of Neurology. Qualifications and guidelines for the physician expert witness. Neurology 2006; 66:13–14. Available at: https://www.aan.com/siteassets/home-page/footer/membership-and-support/member-resources/professionalism–disciplinary-program/05expertwitnessguidelines_ft.pdf. Accessed January 10, 2023.
17. American Academy of Neurology. Disciplinary Action Policy. Available at: https://www.aan.com/siteassets/home-page/footer/membership-and-support/member-resources/professionalism–disciplinary-program/disciplinary-action-policy_revised-2021.pdf. Accessed January 10, 2023.
18. Hutchins JC, Sagsveen MG, Larriviere D. Upholding professionalism – the disciplinary process of the American Academy of Neurology. Neurology 2010;75:2198–203.
19. American Board of Psychiatry and Neurology. Available at: https://www.abpn.com/wp-content/uploads/2022/07/Policy-Regarding-Revocation-of-Certificates_.pdf. Accessed January 10, 2023.
20. Austin v. American Association of Neurological Surgeons, 253 F.3d 967 (7th Cir. 2001).
21. In the United States, some professional organizations maintain copies of depositions and court testimony (e.g., the Defense Research Institute in Chicago; Association of Trial Lawyers of America in Washington D.C.; LexisNexis Collaborative Network for Expert Witness Research; and various medical groups such as the American Association of Neurological Surgeons).

Medical Malpractice and the Neurologist: Specific Neurological Claims

James C. Johnston, MD, JD[a,b],*, Thomas P. Sartwelle, BBA, LLB[c]

KEYWORDS

- Medical malpractice • Neurological malpractice • Negligence • Practice guidelines
- Standard of care • Headache • Cerebrovascular disease • Epilepsy

KEY POINTS

- The most prevalent neurological misadventure is diagnostic error, occurring in one-third to one-half of all claims.
- The most frequent incorrectly diagnosed conditions are malignant neoplasm of the brain, headache (HA), intracranial or intraspinal abscess, nontraumatic subarachnoid hemorrhage, and vertebral fracture.
- These diagnostic errors most commonly stem from failure to perform an adequate history and examination, which is, in fact, the most prevalent procedure resulting in claims against neurologists.
- The most prevalent patient conditions generating recurring suits against neurologists, which affect a large segment of the general population and have the potential for exceptionally high indemnity payments or judgments, may be grouped into HA, cerebrovascular disease, and epilepsy. Recommendations to decrease the risk of a lawsuit are discussed.

INTRODUCTION

The extraordinarily broad scope of neurological malpractice liability precludes a compendium of potential claims. Even limiting claims to diagnostic errors would be overwhelming. Moreover, such a listing would be quickly outdated as emerging diagnostic and therapeutic options open the door for new lawsuits. A more instructive approach is to consider the most prevalent patient conditions generating suits against neurologists. These conditions include, in decreasing frequency, headache, back disorders, occlusion or stenosis of cerebral arteries, convulsions, cerebrovascular accident, migraines, epilepsy, symptoms involving skin and integumentary disorders, displacement of intervertebral disc, and disorders of soft tissue.[1–4]

[a] GlobalNeurology, 17B Farnham Street, Auckland 1052, New Zealand; [b] GlobalNeurology®, 5290 Medical Drive, San Antonio, TX 78229, USA; [c] Hicks Davis Wynn, PC, 3555 Timmons Lane, Suite 1000, Houston, TX 77027, USA
* Corresponding author. 5290 Medical Drive, San Antonio, TX 78229.
E-mail address: johnston@GlobalNeurology.com

Neurol Clin 41 (2023) 493–512
https://doi.org/10.1016/j.ncl.2023.05.002
0733-8619/23/© 2023 Elsevier Inc. All rights reserved.

Back and neck disorders, including intervertebral disc displacement and soft tissue disorders, are not discussed because these claims are generally attributable to straight-forward diagnostic errors, few result in an indemnity payment, and the total indemnity is a small percentage of that paid for all neurology claims.

Risk management strategies are provided for the remaining conditions, arbitrarily grouped together as stroke, epilepsy, and headache (HA), the latter subsuming migraine, brain tumor, and subarachnoid hemorrhage (SAH). Lack of space precludes discussion of the myriad disparate claims involving these conditions. Therefore, several key topics are selected because (1) they affect a large segment of the general population; (2) are frequently seen by neurologists and nonneurologists alike; (3) generate recurring claims; and (4) have the potential for exceptionally high indemnity payments or judgments.

The discussion of each condition is approached from a clinical perspective, with attention to the origin of frequently encountered malpractice claims. It is a format requiring oversimplification of the medical points, which necessitates omitting many conditions, truncating differential diagnoses, and ignoring various diagnostic and therapeutic options. This chapter focuses solely on malpractice issues and is not a substitute for conventional medical writings. Nor is it a treatise of neurological malpractice. It is simply designed to provide a rudimentary understanding of how lawsuits arise and thereby focus discussion on adapting practice patterns to improve patient care and minimize liability risk. References are kept to a minimum and selected to provide the reader with additional background material.

HEADACHE
General Considerations

HAs are ubiquitous, frequently encountered by many physicians, and one of the most common presenting symptoms in malpractice claims against neurologists. HA may be of minimal clinical significance or, paradoxically, herald potentially catastrophic illnesses such as brain tumor, SAH, or meningitis. A complete and accurate diagnosis of the patient with HA requires a detailed history coupled with a full neurological and general medical examination, and possibly diagnostic testing and neuroimaging. The single most important step is to classify the type of HA and simultaneously ascertain whether it is acute, long-standing, or with recent change. This practical approach allows the neurologist to determine the need for any diagnostic testing and initiate a proper treatment plan, all with the appropriate degree of urgency. Too often, the inexperienced, poorly trained, or hurried neurologist either distorts a patient's history or fails to perform an adequate examination, resulting in the wrong diagnosis.

Many malpractice suits stem from the failure to elicit an accurate history, an art that includes the innate ability to establish rapport and instill confidence and trust. The following suggested methodology is presented for the sole purpose of demonstrating several pitfalls that may lead to misdiagnosis. Neurologists should formulate their own techniques, which will evolve with time, experience, and continuing education.

- Allow ample time for the consultation. Introduce yourself and invite the patient to sit for an interview before changing into a gown. Advise the patient that you have read the referral letter but never accept either the patient's or referring physician's diagnosis.
- "Tell me about your HAs." Allow the patient to speak uninterruptedly before asking questions. Then begin open-ended queries to determine the quality, severity, location, duration, and time course of events, as well as precipitating, exacerbating, and relieving factors. It is helpful to ask the patient to describe a

particular attack. Determine whether the patient has more than one type of HA. It is essential to separately evaluate each HA type, even if this requires subsequent appointments due to time constraints.

- Communication skills and understanding the cultural context are critical. Knowing which clues to follow and when to interrupt the patient are fundamental to an accurate history. Failure to understand the patient's terminology may lead to misdiagnosis, for example, translating the word "throbbing" to migraine. It is not uncommon for an HA specialist to distort the history until it fits a preconceived diagnostic category.
- The scope of the history must be sufficiently broad to address systemic diseases that may be relevant to the HA. Past, family, social, and travel histories provide valuable information. It is often enlightening to solicit the patient's opinion regarding the cause of HA.

Specific Approach

Evaluation requires a systematic approach to exclude more serious conditions, diagnose the primary HA, and formulate a treatment plan. There are particular aspects of each step that seem to generate recurring claims. This overview is limited to nontraumatic HAs in the adult population, with particular attention to the more common diagnostic and treatment errors.

First step

The first step is to exclude serious conditions causing secondary HAs; it is complicated because primary and secondary HAs may share similar clinical presentations. The differential diagnosis is exceedingly long, and each case must be evaluated on an individual basis. The neurologist should be attentive to warning signs or "red flags" suggesting a secondary HA and proceed with appropriate diagnostic and therapeutic interventions. The authors use the mnemonic "SIGNAL" to highlight the most misdiagnosed secondary HAs:

Sudden-onset (thunderclap) HA;
Increasing or changing HA;
Generalized disease with HA;
Neurological or focal signs with HA;
Activity, exertion, or cough HA; and
Labor, pregnancy, or postpartum HA.

Sudden-onset (thunderclap) headache. The sudden onset of severe HA mandates immediate and thorough evaluation for potential causes, including SAH, intracerebral hemorrhage, venous or sinus thrombosis, intracranial or extracranial arterial dissection, aneurysmal expansion, pituitary apoplexy, ischemic stroke, reversible cerebral vasoconstriction syndrome, spontaneous intracranial hypotension, and less common conditions.[5–8] Most of the nontraumatic SAH cases (85%) are due to saccular aneurysmal hemorrhage; 5% due to arteriovenous malformation; and the remainder with a negative arteriogram are divided between benign perimesencephalic hemorrhage and rare etiopathogenetic mechanisms.[9]

The misdiagnosis or failure to diagnose SAH consistently results in a high percentage of paid claims with a high total indemnity, as expected with 50% mortality and significant morbidity, and there are significantly fewer claims involving the complex management of SAH.[10,11] Most cases center on a failure to recognize the broad spectrum of clinical presentations, failure to order or understand the limitations of computerized tomography (CT), or failure to perform a lumbar puncture (LP) or properly interpret the results.[12–14]

The *sine qua non* of SAH is a sudden HA classically described as the "first" or "worst HA of my life," which may be unilateral, associated with nausea or vomiting and followed by signs of meningeal irritation. The word "sudden" in this context cannot be overemphasized. Perhaps a better description is that the HA presents with maximal severity at onset. There may be cognitive impairment, focal deficits, or, in up to one-half of cases, a history of premonitory symptoms suggestive of a sentinel bleed or aneurysmal expansion. The clinical presentation is variable, and diagnosis requires a high index of suspicion: half of the patients present as Hunt Hess grade I (minimal HA) or II (moderate to severe HA, no deficit except cranial nerve palsy); 10% have no HA at onset; 8% describe a slowly increasing HA; and a stiff neck is absent in 36% of patients.[15–19] The known migraineur presenting with a sentinel HA may be misdiagnosed as having breakthrough symptoms; a thorough history is helpful, as many patients recognize that the HA is different from a "usual migraine."[20,21] In the absence of a clear history, it is always better to investigate a migraine than risk missing an SAH.

The patient with thunderclap HA must have an immediate brain CT, which is most sensitive for SAH in the first 6 hours, and then rapidly diminishes by 3 days after the initial event, with sensitivity decaying to 50% or less by 1 week post-ictus.[22–25] Magnetic resonance (MR) imaging with gradient-recalled echo (GRE) or fluid-attenuated inversion recovery (FLAIR) pulse sequences provides excellent sensitivity in acute hemorrhage, but the value is limited by practical difficulties including accessibility, and further refinement is warranted for the use in subacute and chronic stages.[26,27]

If a timely CT is negative, it is essential to perform LP with measurement of opening pressure and testing for xanthochromia, which may take up to 12 hours posthemorrhage to develop and will remain for up to 2 weeks.[28] Xanthochromia, by visual inspection, carries an approximate 70% likelihood of a ruptured aneurysm, with a 93% sensitivity, 95% specificity, and 99% negative predictive value; spectrophotometry is complementary when visual inspection is negative for xanthochromia.[29] Other causes of yellow discolored cerebrospinal fluid (CSF) must not be ignored (eg, jaundice, rifampin, hypercarotenemia, elevated CSF protein, traumatic tap).

Further evaluation based on the clinical presentation, as well as CT and LP results, may warrant cerebral angiography or MR imaging as well as neurosurgical consultation for definite intervention.[30] The timing of surgery, if indicated, is critical for an operable aneurysm, and failure to expeditiously arrange care would be regarded as negligent.

The management of blood pressure, glucose, cardiopulmonary status, hemodynamics, seizures, and prevention and treatment of delayed cerebral ischemia are complex and certainly give rise to malpractice claims, but the limits of this chapter preclude discussion because the number of these claims is proportionately minor compared with misdiagnosis or failure to diagnose SAH and, for the surgeons, operative misadventure or poor outcome.

There may be a question of whether further investigation is necessary in a patient with severe, sudden HA, who has a normal neurological examination, normal CT, and normal CSF studies. In 1 retrospective and 4 prospective studies of patients with this presentation, none suffered subsequent hemorrhage or sudden death.[31–35] Thus, angiography may not be necessary in most patients with a normal CT and CSF analysis. If the CT is negative but LP positive, then CT angiography is necessary. Further imaging may be required depending on the clinical picture, and as always thorough documentation is warranted.

Increasing, escalating, or worsening headache. The patient's HA pattern must be interpreted considering the overall history. Recent onset HAs with progression may indicate a tumor, subdural hematoma, or other intra-axial or extra-axial mass lesion, and focal deficits may be present. A slow growing mass may not be associated with any neurological deficits. The differential also includes sphenoid sinusitis, venous sinus thrombosis, or meningitis. Chronic primary HAs with progression may represent the development of a new, superimposed HA disorder (primary or secondary) or transformation of the primary disorder. It may be impossible to clinically distinguish the transformed migraine, often precipitated by medication overuse, from a new HA disorder. Thus, the presentation of an escalating HA, whether acute or chronic, warrants investigation.

Generalized or systemic disease with headache. There are myriad systemic diseases presenting with acute HA including intracranial (eg, meningitis, encephalitis, sphenoid sinusitis) and generalized (eg, Lyme disease, syphilis) infections; neoplasm including paraneoplastic disease and leptomeningeal metastases; vascular conditions; autoimmune disorders; metabolic diseases; and toxic exposures. The diagnosis requires proficient examination with attention to systemic signs serving to guide diagnostic intervention. For example, the older patient with HA and visual symptoms may require temporal artery biopsy for giant cell arteritis.

Neurological or focal signs with headache. HA associated with transient or permanent focal deficits, other than a typical aura, may be due to intracranial structural disease and requires further evaluation. Although this point seems straightforward, delay or failure to diagnose brain tumor remains one of the most common errors in neurology. It is difficult to understand why, especially given the advances in neuroimaging over the past 3 decades. Perhaps the sheer volume of HAs leads to an apathetic approach, or it may simply reflect the inimitable presentation of many intracranial tumors—they generally do not have dramatic characteristics. In fact, brain tumor patients may present with isolated HA.[36] Although HA is the most consistent symptom of an intracranial tumor, it often meets the International Headache Society criteria for tension-type, migraine, or mixed HA.[37,38] HA due to supratentorial tumors, such as a nondominant frontal mass, may cause psychological symptoms with minimal or absent physical features, leading to inappropriate psychiatric referral. Certain brain tumors mimic primary HA syndromes—a pituitary tumor presenting as migraine or SUNCT.[39–41] Additional subtle warning signs of a tumor may be overlooked: a change in HA pattern; chronic HA with new symptoms; new-onset HA after age 50 years; HA in children or the elderly; and HA with Valsalva maneuver. Tumor-related symptoms may simply be unrecognized or their significance unappreciated for months or years. Whatever the reason, more aggressive imaging is necessary to ensure patients with tumor-related HAs are diagnosed without undue delay.[42,43]

Activity or cough-related headache. HAs triggered by cough, exertion, or sexual activity are frequently associated with posterior fossa structural abnormalities and warrant MR imaging for a definitive diagnosis. In one analysis, 42% of patients with cough HA harbored intracranial pathology; in another study more than 10% had structural lesions, predominantly in the posterior fossa.[44–46]

Labor-, pregnancy-, or postpartum-related headache. The new onset of HAs or progression of known primary HAs during pregnancy or postpartum raises the concern of sinus thrombosis, cerebral infarction, carotid dissection, pituitary apoplexy, and preeclampsia. These disorders most commonly occur during the third trimester or postpartum, present with HA, and may be associated with focal signs or seizures.

Second step

The second step, after excluding secondary HAs, is to diagnose the primary HA in accordance with International Classification of Headache Disorders criteria.[47,48] It is beyond the scope of this writing to review the various HA syndromes; however, the importance of correctly diagnosing the patient cannot be overstated. Too often the neurologist incorrectly labels the HA type during initial consultation and, despite a poor response to treatment, never reconsiders the diagnosis, creating a breeding ground for malpractice claims.

Third step

The third step is to treat primary HA with a comprehensive multimodality approach incorporating pharmacological intervention predicated on evidence-based guidelines. Management strategies for acute and chronic HA are detailed in the literature, and each therapeutic modality is subject to a unique array of claims. A significant number of these suits allege medication errors, examples including failure to manage rebound phenomena, inappropriate use of medications, failure to properly monitor medication, and failure to identify side effects. It is important to recognize when to use acute or prophylactic therapy, document the reasons for that decision and, if initiating prophylactic coverage, and choose a drug with the highest benefit to risk ratio, with the fewest side effects, and ideally a medication that also treats any coexisting disease. Other medication-related suits may be avoided by starting a drug at the lowest effective dose, slowly titrating until maximal benefits are achieved or side effects supervene, providing an adequate trial before changing medications, performing appropriate monitoring, and tapering off at the proper time.

Refractory Headache

Patients with refractory HA may be misdiagnosed or improperly treated due to an incomplete or incorrect diagnosis (ie, misdiagnosed primary HA; undiagnosed secondary HA, including failure to recognize that migraineurs may suffer secondary HAs; or failure to recognize multiple HA types); improper imaging studies; ignoring exacerbating factors or triggers; poor pharmacotherapeutic management; or neglecting rebound phenomena.

Neuroimaging in the Patient with Headache

The role of neuroimaging in the adult patient with HA and a normal neurological examination remains a highly controversial topic.

The American Headache Society Practice Guidelines for neuroimaging in HA state that "[t]here is no necessity to do neuroimaging in patients with headaches consistent with migraine who have a normal neurologic examination, and there are no atypical features or red flags present."[49,50] These parameters reiterate prior guidelines, based on outdated studies plagued by serious methodological flaws and limitations that underestimated the prevalence of significant intracranial abnormalities in patients with HA and a normal neurological examination; by way of example, one-quarter of patients with biopsy-proven brain tumor presented with an incidental lesion, nonspecific findings, or isolated HA.[51]

Arguments against imaging because of the possibility of incidental findings are untenable. The harm of missing a brain tumor or other structural lesion outweighs any concern of uncovering an incidental finding. In addition, some of these findings are mislabeled incidental and warrant treatment (eg, arachnoid cysts), monitoring (eg, aneurysm), or further evaluation (eg, stroke). The patient should at least be given the option of proceeding with imaging after a frank discussion of the facts, which is the basic tenet of informed consent.

But the most common diagnostic error in neurology, year after year, is to label a patient with migraine or other HA disorder in the absence of neuroimaging, only to find that subsequent evaluation uncovers a brain tumor or other structural lesion. In the case of a malignant glioma, a delay may not make any significant difference to the patient's ultimate fate. In contrast, any delay in diagnosing a benign tumor increases operative risk, affecting mortality and postoperative morbidity. Arguments that earlier diagnosis would not have materially affected the outcome are generally unsuccessful. There may be absolutely no relationship between the HA and brain tumor or other structural lesion, but the trier of fact will likely find otherwise if the neurologist failed to order a timely imaging study. Thus, the decision to forego neuroimaging in a patient with HAs requires a great deal of experience and clinical acumen. For many neurologists, it would simply be prudent to perform an imaging study on every patient with HA early in the evaluation. Of course, there is no reason to repeat a test if already performed, assuming no change in the patient's condition.

MR imaging is the imaging procedure of choice for evaluation of secondary HA, relegating CT to the limited role of excluding intracranial blood such as in SAH or detecting skull fractures or bone disease.[52] MR imaging is the superior choice in most circumstances due to its sensitivity to venous thrombosis, extracranial hematomas, neoplasms, white matter abnormalities, and meningeal disease as well as its ability to visualize the posterior fossa, cervicomedullary junction, and pituitary region, while avoiding radiation exposure.

The neurologist must be familiar with the correct MR imaging sequences to order (eg, T2, FLAIR, GRE, diffusion-weighted imaging, MR angiography, and so forth), when to use gadolinium, and the proper imaging views, all based on the presumptive diagnosis or disorder. Equally important is the ability to recognize subtle abnormalities that may be reflective of a particular disorder. For example, increased optic nerve sheath diameter may indicate idiopathic intracranial hypertension as the cause of a secondary HA.

Unfortunately, American neurologists may be deterred from ordering these studies due to managed care constraints and misguided information from "Choosing Wisely" and related organizations. Therefore, failure to diagnose brain tumor will likely remain one of the most common malpractice claims.

CEREBROVASCULAR DISEASE
General Considerations

Globally, 6 million people die from stroke each year; it is the fourth leading cause of death in the United States with almost 800,000 strokes annually.[53] The development of specific treatment options (thrombolysis; endovascular therapy) and refinement of prevention strategies (anticoagulation; carotid endarterectomy), along with improved diagnostic modalities, creates a heightened expectation of proper stroke management and, combined with the catastrophic impact of stroke, portends increasing litigation in this area. The following clinical scenarios leading to common malpractice claims include some background references and guidelines, but keep in mind that for any claim, the standard of care is based on the prevailing practice at the time of the incident.

Thrombolytic Therapy

Recombinant tissue plasminogen activator (rtPA) thrombolysis represents the neurological standard of care for acute ischemic stroke,[54,55] and although a significant percentage of eligible patients do not receive the drug because of transportation, geographic location, hospital capabilities, and a few other reasons, it should be administered within 4.5 hours after stroke onset in eligible patients, with strict adherence to the protocol inclusion and exclusion criteria.[56–64] Tenecteplase may replace alteplase due in part to ease of administration and lower incidence in intracerebral hemorrhage and will probably have a similar liability profile, but in the absence of any legal cases the following discussion is limited to rtPA.[65]

The failure to recommend or administer rtPA to an eligible patient may constitute negligence unless it can be proved that rtPA would not have made a material difference in the patient's outcome. The neurologist deciding not to use rtPA in an acute ischemic stroke is at a high risk for claims and should clearly document the reasons for that decision in the medical records. One recurring error is the administration of anticoagulants or antiplatelet agents during the first 24 hours after rtPA administration, which increases the risk of hemorrhage. It is important for the neurologist to resist pressure from the emergency physician or family to use rtPA unless the patient meets all inclusion and exclusion criteria. Modification of the criteria, especially the time constraint, decreases the benefit and increases the risk of intracerebral hemorrhage. It is, therefore, crucial to determine the time of stroke onset. A common error is labeling the onset as the time symptoms were first observed rather than the last time the patient was known to be well. For example, if the patient awakens with deficits, then the onset time is considered the time the patient went to bed, not when the symptoms were first noticed on wakening. The same holds true for patients unable to communicate these details. Likewise, patients with stroke-related neglect syndromes cannot reliably observe the onset time. Again, it is imperative to follow the guidelines. But note that recent studies indicate select patients have a better functional outcome when treated with rtPA for a "wake up" stroke[66] - this provides an example of the many scenarios where a neurologist may consider all the risks and benefits and decide it is in the patient's best interest to deviate from the protocol. This decision should be discussed with the patient or legal representative and family and thoroughly documented in the records.

The failure to obtain valid informed consent may precipitate a malpractice action separate from negligence. Informed consent mandates a frank discussion regarding the benefits and risks of tPA, including the potential for hemorrhage, coma, and death. The acute stroke patient may not be able to fully participate in the process due to communication deficits or cognitive impairment. Options should then be discussed with a close family member and documented, but only a legal representative (guardian or person with written power of attorney) can give consent. If the patient is unable to give consent and no legal representative is available, the neurologist may proceed with tPA when it is the most reasonable option. Courts recognize implied consent; there is an assumption that a competent individual would have agreed to the procedure.[67,68]

Endovascular Therapy

Endovascular therapy is the treatment of choice in patients with acute ischemic stroke and proximal anterior circulation large vessel occlusion if there are limited signs of early ischemic changes on neuroimaging, the patient can be treated within 6 hours of stroke symptom onset, using a second-generation stent retriever or a catheter aspiration device, and regardless of whether the patient received rtPA.[69] Two clinical trials demonstrated excellent clinical outcomes in patients treated up to 24 hours after the onset of stroke symptoms.[70,71] The specific criteria for intervention are relatively well defined at this time, but since outcomes depend on the interaction of several variables including age, infarct volume, and functional status, combined with beneficial effects of an expanded time window in select patients, along with variations based on specific procedures, the future of endovascular therapy will continue to evolve and remain an area ripe for litigation.

Anticoagulation Therapy

The immediate use of anticoagulation for preventing recurrent stroke after an acute ischemic infarction, fluctuating basilar artery thrombosis, or imminent carotid occlusion or other noncardioembolic indication remains controversial despite an absence of supporting evidence, making it increasingly difficult to defend hemorrhagic complications.[72,73] Warfarin or direct oral anticoagulants may be beneficial in the early period after an ischemic event but there is no definitive evidence that long-term anticoagulation for thrombosis or embolism outweighs the potential risks except in certain patients with nonvalvular atrial fibrillation (NVAF), prosthetic heart valves, acute myocardial infarction, specific valvular heart diseases, mechanical left ventricular assist devices, and a few other conditions.[74]

NVAF significantly increases the risk of stroke across all age groups, aggravated by high-risk factors (hypertension, diabetes mellitus, left ventricular dysfunction, transient ischemic attack [TIA] or prior stroke), and anticoagulation is the accepted standard of care in eligible patients based on risk stratification.[75–77] For patients with a stroke or TIA in the setting of NVAF, it is reasonable to initiate anticoagulation early unless there is a high risk of hemorrhagic conversion. If anticoagulation is contraindicated, or the patient is at low risk of stroke, then antiplatelet therapy may be the most appropriate treatment.[78]

The use of warfarin is complicated by the risk of bleeding, or, conversely, if the dose is too low then a subsequent stroke may lead to claim that proper anticoagulation would have prevented the event. There are significant potential complications, serious interactions with numerous other medications, and the pharmacokinetics are difficult to manage, leading to a broad source of claims, which may be partially mitigated by enlisting an anticoagulant management service.

The newer anticoagulants (eg, rivaroxaban, dabigatran, apixaban) are preferable in most cases and have the advantages of fixed dosing, fewer drug interactions, and no need for laboratory monitoring.[79–83] However, warfarin may remain the drug of choice for patients with renal impairment or liver disease, or an anticipated need for anticoagulation reversal, although this relative contraindication may change with the recent availability of reversal agents for dabigatran and factor Xa inhibitors.

The reasons for or against anticoagulating a patient at risk should be documented in the medical records. For example, if the increased risk of bleeding due to gait instability outweighs the potential benefits of anticoagulation, then careful documentation may protect against litigation if the patient suffers a massive embolus. Patient and family education concerning the management of anticoagulation is crucial and should be clearly documented.

Antiplatelet Therapy

Antiplatelet therapy is the preferred treatment of secondary stroke prevention in patients with symptomatic intracranial atherosclerotic disease.[84] Dual antiplatelet therapy, when initiated soon after a high-risk TIA or minor stroke, and continued for 21 to 90 days, is more effective than single antiplatelet therapy in reducing recurrent ischemic stroke; and there may be some benefit to cilostazol, but as always the risk of hemorrhage must be weighed against potential benefits of dual therapy.[85,86] Aspirin monotherapy or the combination of extended release dipyridamole plus aspirin may be indicated in the chronic phase after TIA or ischemic stroke; clopidogrel monotherapy may be considered especially in patients unable to tolerate aspirin, but there are contradictory recommendations, variations, and limitations with changing guidelines.[87] And the clinical management is more complicated than this oversimplification, with individualized considerations affecting medication choices, management of modifiable risk factors, addressing rehabilitation including minimizing the risk of falls, and other issues that may lead to a lawsuit. Failure to provide antiplatelet therapy may precipitate a suit if the patient suffers a cerebral infarction, and conversely, there may be liability for the patient older than 60 years suffering a hemorrhage due to the use of aspirin. Again, these concerns serve as a reminder to document clinical decision-making. From a broader legal perspective, and perhaps more common, the neurologist and primary physician may be sued for failure to evaluate TIAs in a timely fashion.

Carotid Endarterectomy and Carotid Angioplasty (Stenting)

Carotid endarterectomy (CEA) significantly reduces the incidence of cerebral infarction in select patients with high-grade carotid stenosis (70%–99% diameter reduction), is moderately useful for symptomatic patients with 50% to 69% stenosis based on specific patient factors, is not indicated for symptomatic patients with less than 50% stenosis, and individualized decisions are required for the smaller benefit in asymptomatic patients with 60% to 99% stenosis.[88–92] There must be careful patient selection with attention to physiological factors (eg, age, congestive heart failure, coronary heart disease, low ejection fraction, and similar concerns) and anatomic features (eg, high-grade tandem lesions in the ipsilateral intracranial arteries, bilateral carotid stenosis, or severe contralateral carotid artery stenosis or occlusion), and skill of the surgical team is paramount, as intervention is only recommended if estimated perioperative morbidity and mortality is less than 6%.[93]

The most common malpractice claims are failure to diagnose TIA or minor stroke and failure to evaluate for carotid stenosis, leading to a recurrent or massive stroke. Every patient with a TIA or stroke should have appropriate vascular imaging unless surgery is plainly contraindicated. Most patients with symptomatic carotid artery stenosis greater than 70% should be offered CEA or carotid angioplasty. Other degrees of stenosis require individualized considerations that must be well documented. Delay in referring a symptomatic patient with high-grade stenosis for definitive treatment may precipitate a negligence claim if the patient suffers a subsequent stroke, which is more likely soon after the initial event.

Surgery, if indicated, should be offered soon after a TIA or nondisabling stroke, preferably within 2 weeks of the last symptomatic event, but following a moderate to severe stroke it may be appropriate to delay CEA for 4 to 6 weeks due to the risk of hemorrhagic conversion.[94] Carotid stenting is still evolving from a liability perspective but there are situations suggesting preference over CEA including certain anatomic features (high carotid bifurcation; severe cervical spondylosis) and specific clinical scenarios (contralateral carotid occlusion; previous radical neck surgery or radiation to the neck; recurrent stenosis after endarterectomy; significant cardiac or severe pulmonary disease).[95,96]

EPILEPSY
General Considerations

Epilepsy affects more than 3 million adults and children in the United States.[97–99] Approximately 150,000 adults will present annually with a first seizure, with almost half recurring to be classified as epilepsy; the lifetime cumulative risk of a seizure ranges from 8% to 10%, with a 3% chance of developing epilepsy.[100] These disorders present formidable legal challenges due to the variable clinical symptoms, diverse etiopathogenetic mechanisms, and diagnostic and therapeutic complexity in patients who commonly harbor intellectual impairment, cognitive dysfunction, and psychiatric symptoms.[101,102]

Driving

Every US state restricts issuance of a driver's license to individuals who have suffered loss of consciousness. The laws differ among states but generally require that an individual be seizure free for a period of time, varying from no specified duration to 1 year, certified by a physician, before obtaining a license. Neurologists are rightfully concerned about potential liability when certifying that a patient with epilepsy is capable of driving. Some states grant immunity, although the level varies among jurisdictions, ranging from "good faith" immunity to immunity from suit. In other states, physicians are not granted statutory immunity from liability for the information they provide to the state or for damages arising out of a seizure-related accident. In states without physician immunity laws, courts may still refuse to impose liability on the neurologist who exercised reasonable care and good faith in reporting to the state.

Most states have voluntary reporting statues; 6—California, Delaware, Nevada, New Jersey, Oregon, and Pennsylvania—have express mandatory reporting statutes requiring physicians to report patients with epilepsy (or other disorders associated with loss of consciousness or impaired ability to drive).[103] The neurological standard of care for reporting the epileptic patient varies according to the laws and regulations of each state. It is incumbent on neurologists to know the relevant statutes in their jurisdiction and understand the common law trends for any ambiguous issues. The neurologist has a duty to advise patients of the legislation in their particular state, as well as a duty to emphasize the importance of complying with the law. If the state has an explicit self-reporting requirement, patients should be advised in writing to comply, retaining a copy of the letter in the medical records. The discussion of driving restrictions as well as restrictions on other activities, the effect of discontinuing or reducing dosage of a drug, and possible side effects of medications in relation to driving should be clearly documented in the records. These issues should be reiterated and documented on any medication change, due to the increased risk of breakthrough seizures.

If an epileptic patient continues driving because the neurologist failed to report where reporting is mandatory or failed to instruct the patient in a voluntary reporting state, then a seizure-related accident may trigger a malpractice suit by the patient or patient's estate. Therefore, it is imperative that the neurologist clearly document patient instructions in the medical records and keep a copy of any notification sent to the state. The patient who drives against medical advice is a special concern, as *Tarasoff* reasoning may be imputed to the neurologist who advises a patient not to drive, learns the patient continues driving, and fails to take further action.[104] In this situation, the neurologist should inform the patient in writing about the potential consequences of driving and consider filing a voluntary report with the appropriate state agency. There may be statutory protection for a voluntary report made in good faith and consistent with the prevailing standard of care. However, the level of protection varies among jurisdictions, making it advisable to consult legal counsel.

Neurologists may be liable to third parties for failing to report a patient or certifying a patient to drive; this is an emerging area of liability, and most decisions turn on whether the neurologist owes a duty to the third party. Courts have ruled in both directions, and the issue remains far from settled. Neurologists should adapt practice patterns to comport with the relevant legal trends in their jurisdiction, but even third-party liability is minimized by effective patient discussions, proper reporting, and thorough documentation.

Teratogenesis

There are more than one-half million women with epilepsy of childbearing age in the United States; 3 to 5 births per thousand are to epileptic women.[105,106] Epilepsy is a common neurological disorder in pregnancy and raises a host of legal and medical issues. The most serious concern is the potential for congenital malformations in the offspring of mothers taking antiepileptic drugs (AEDs). These mothers have an up to 9% risk of bearing a child with congenital malformations, 3-fold higher than nonepileptic mothers.[107] This higher risk is probably multifactorial, with genetic and social components, but AEDs are clearly implicated as human teratogens, well recognized across multiple registries including the North American Antiepileptic Drug Pregnancy Registry (NAAEDPR), the UK and Ireland Epilepsy Pregnancy Register, and the Australian Pregnancy Register.[108]

In general, AEDs taken during the first trimester share an increased risk of major congenital malformations, which commonly include orofacial clefts, congenital heart disease, neural tube defects, and urogenital malformations.[109] In 2022, the American Academy of Neurology reaffirmed evidence-based practice parameters on management of women with epilepsy, which provided the limited but important conclusions that valproic acid (VPA) exposure during the first trimester is associated with midline defects at a rate of 6% to 9% and reduced cognitive outcomes; monotherapy exposure to phenytoin or phenobarbital possibly reduces cognitive outcomes; and polytherapy compared to monotherapy is associated with an increased risk of birth defects and reduced cognitive outcomes.[110–113]

Subsequently, a number of large, worldwide pregnancy registries have substantiated these findings and provided significant additional information allowing refinement of treatment recommendations.[114–121] Additional data on the AEDs continues to emerge and mandates close follow-up on a regular basis. The available information at this time suggests that lamotrigine, oxcarbazepine, and levetiracetam are probably the safest AEDs, whereas valproate, phenobarbital, phenytoin, carbamazepine, and topiramate should be avoided. All AEDs probably have a dose-related risk of major congenital malformations, and a family history of major congenital malformations will increase the risk with AED exposure.[122]

Malpractice suits for AED-induced fetal malformations have the potential for extraordinarily large settlements or judgments, and tolling of the statute of limitations is commonplace. The neurologist must address a variety of complex issues in epileptic women who take AEDs during their reproductive years in order to minimize liability for these claims. The recent guidelines are hampered by a paucity of evidence limiting the recommendations, so the following suggestions focus on some of the clinical points commonly raised in lawsuits.[123–125]

Detailed counseling early in the reproductive years should include a discussion of the increased risk of seizures during pregnancy, importance of medication compliance, necessity of regular follow-up with AED levels, risk of malformations, folic acid and vitamin K supplementation, and the importance of avoiding coteratogens. Before pregnancy, it is important to determine whether AEDs are necessary; for example, if the patient is receiving an anticonvulsant for migraine, depression, pain, or some other disorder, it may be possible to discontinue the drug. In addition, if the patient with a single type of seizure has been in remission for 2 to 5 years, has a normal neurological examination, and no electroencephalogram abnormalities, then it may be reasonable to gradually withdraw the drug. The taper must be performed slowly over months, and completed at least 6 months before conception, as seizure recurrence is most likely during this time.

If treatment is indicated, every effort should be made to place the patient on monotherapy with the lowest effective dose of the most suitable AED. Frequent daily dosing will avoid high peak levels, possibly reducing the potential for teratogenesis. There are several other nuances that must be considered on a case-by-case basis with careful balancing of myriad factors. For example, a low-dose polytherapy may be safer than select high-dose monotherapy in certain cases, considering factors such as seizure type, potential harm, psychological profile, and individual health concerns. The AED levels should be monitored at least preconception, at the beginning of each trimester, the last month of pregnancy, and 2 months post-partum. Pregnancy screening should include serum alpha-fetoprotein at 16 to 18 weeks and a level II ultrasound at 18 to 20 weeks. If indicated, amniocentesis may be offered at 18 to 20 weeks. The patient should be properly counseled if there is a serious malformation and provided with the option to terminate the pregnancy. The administration of folic acid in the early stages of pregnancy may decrease the incidence of congenital malformations including neural tube defects and, despite the limited guideline recommendations, should be given to all women of childbearing potential.[126–128] Optimal dosage for women with epilepsy remains controversial, and data must be extrapolated from nonepileptic women, with most organizations advising 0.4 mg to 4.0 mg daily. It is a matter of clinical judgment, the authors recommending 4.0 mg daily until at least 12 weeks gestational age (noting 5 mg or more daily may raise concerns), and this dose seems affirmed by the American College of Obstetrics and Gynecology.[129]

It is not uncommon for women with epilepsy to present to the neurologist after becoming pregnant. In general, the risk of uncontrolled epilepsy is greater than the risk of AED-induced teratogenesis; thus, drug treatment must be continued throughout pregnancy. For several reasons, it is a serious albeit common error to change medications for the sole purpose of reducing teratogenic risk. First, there is a risk of precipitating seizures that may reduce placental blood flow and impair fetal oxygenation. Second, the critical period of organogenesis has usually passed, and discontinuing an AED does not lower the risk of congenital malformations. For example, neural tube closure occurs during gestation weeks 3 to 4; by the time most women recognize pregnancy it is probably too late to avoid related malformations by adjusting AEDs. Third, exposing the fetus to a second agent during the crossover period is akin to polytherapy and increases the teratogenic risk. Thus, if an epileptic woman presents after conception on effective monotherapy, the AED should generally be continued although changing drugs must be considered with VPA, phenobarbital, or topiramate. Hemorrhagic disease of the newborn may occur in neonates exposed to hepatic enzyme inducing AEDs and requires special attention including maternal administration of oral vitamin K during the last month of pregnancy.

Portions of the text are updated from James C. Johnston, Neurological malpractice and non-malpractice liability, Neurol Clin 2010; 28(2):441 to 458, with permission.

AUTHOR CONTRIBUTIONS

The authors contributed equally to the research, development, writing, review, and approval of the content.

DECLARATION OF CONFLICTING INTERESTS

The authors declared no potential conflicts of interest with respect to the research, authorship, and publication of this article.

FUNDING

The authors received no financial support for the research, authorship, and publication of this article.

REFERENCES

1. Martin KL. Medscape Neurologist Malpractice Report 2019. Available at: https://www.medscape.com/slideshow/2019-malpractice-report-neuro-6012448. (Accessed December 12, 2022).
2. Physicians Insurers Association of America. Risk management review (neurology). Rockville, MD: PIAA; 2013.
3. See also aon/ASHMR hospital and physician liability benchmark analysis 2021.
4. Physicians Insurers Association of America. Risk management review (neurology). Rockville, MD: PIAA; 2009.
5. Etminan N, Macdonald RL. Management of aneurysmal subarachnoid hemorrhage. In: Wijdicks EFM, Kramer AH, editors. Handbook of Clin Neurol, 140. Amsterdam): Elsevier; 2017. p. 195–228.
6. Chou SH. Subarachnoid hemorrhage. Continuum (Minneap Minn) 2021;27(5):1201–45.
7. See also MacDonald RL, Schweizer TA. Spontaneous subarachnoid hemorrhage. Lancet 2017;389:655–66.
8. Muehischlegel S, Kursun O, Topcuoglu MA, et al. Differentiating reversible cerebral vasoconstriction syndrome from other causes of subarachnoid hemorrhage. JAMA Neurol 2013;70(10):1254–60.
9. Supra notes 5, 6.
10. van Gijn J, Kerr RS, Rinkel GJ. Subarachnoid hemorrhage. Lancet 2007;369(9558):306–18.
11. Supra note 2, Physicians Insurers Association of America. Risk Management Review (Neurology) at vi.
12. Supra note 2 Etminan N, Macdonald RL. See also, Mayer PL, Awad IA, Todor R, et al. Misdiagnosis of symptomatic cerebral aneurysm. Prevalence and correlation with outcome at four institutions. Stroke 1996;27:1558–63.
13. Oh S, Lim YC, Shim YS, et al. Initial misdiagnosis of aneurysmal subarachnoid hemorrhage: associating factors and its prognosis. Acta Neurochir 2018;160(6):1105–13.
14. Kowalski RG, Claassen J, Kreiter KT. Initial misdiagnosis and outcome after subarachnoid hemorrhage. JAMA 2004;291(7):866–9.
15. Maher M, Schweizer, Macdonald RL. Treatment of spontaneous subarachnoid hemorrhage. Stroke 2020;51:1326–32.
16. Interventional neuroradiology. In: Hetts SW, Cooke DL, editors. Handbook of Clin Neurol, 176. Amsterdam): Elsevier; 2021. p. 2–427.
17. See Weir B. Headache from aneurysms. Cephalalgia 1994;14(2):79–87.
18. See also Linn FHH, Rinkel GJE, Algra A, et al. Headache characteristics in subarachnoid hemorrhage and benign thunderclap headache. J Neuro Neurosurg Psychiatry 1998;65:791–3.
19. See van Gijn J, Rinkel GJE. Subarachnoid hemorrhage: diagnosis, causes and management. Brain 2001;124(2):249–78.
20. Supra note 7. See Suarez JI, Tarr RW, Selman WR. Aneurysmal subarachnoid hemorrhage. NEJM 2006;354(4):387–96.
21. See also Brisman JL, Song JK, Newell DW. Cerebral aneurysms. NEJM 2006;355(9):928–39.

22. Supra note 8 Perry JJ, Stiell IG, Sivilotti ML, et al. Sensitivity of computed tomography performed within six hours of onset of headache for diagnosis of subarachnoid hemorrhage: prospective cohort study. BMJ 2011;343:d4277.
23. van Gijn J, van Dongen KJ. The time course of aneurysmal hemorrhage on computed tomograms. Neurorad 1982;23(3):153–6.
24. Edlow JA. Diagnosis of subarachnoid hemorrhage. Neurocrit Care 2005;2: 99–109.
25. de Oliveria MAL, Mansur A, Murphy A, et al. Aneurysmal subarachnoid hemorrhage from a neuroimaging perspective. Crit Care 2014;18(6):557.
26. Id Nelson SE, Sair HI, Stevens RD. Magnetic resonance imaging in aneurysmal subarachnoid hemorrhage: current evidence and future directions. Neurocrit Care 2018;29:241–52.
27. Mohamed M, Heasly DC, Yagmurla DM. Fluid associated inversion recovery MR imaging and subarachnoid hemorrhage: not a panacea. Am J Neurorad 2004; 25:545–50.
28. Supra notes 15-19. See also Stewart H, Reuben A and McDonald J. LP or not LP, that is the question: gold standard or unnecessary procedure in subarachnoid hemorrhage, *Emerg Med J*, 31 (9), 2014, 720–723.
29. Supra notes 15-19. See also Petzold A, Keir G and Sharpe TL. Why human color vision cannot reliably detect cerebrospinal fluid xanthochromia, *Stroke*, 36 (6), 2005, 1295–1297.
30. Supra notes 15-19. See also Guidelines for the management of aneurysmal subarachnoid hemorrhage: A guideline for healthcare professionals from the American Heart Association/American Stroke Association, *Stroke*, 43, 2012, 1711–1737, Available at: https://www.ahajournals.org/doi/pdf/10.1161/STR.0b013e3182587 839, Accessed January 19, 2023. [Note: The pending 2023 Guideline for the Management of Patients with Aneurysmal Subarachnoid Hemorrage will replace the 2012 Guideline].
31. Wijdicks EFM, Kerkhoff H, van Gijn J. Long term follow up of 71 patients with thunderclap headache mimicking subarachnoid hemorrhage. Lancet 1988; 2(8602):68–9.
32. Harling DW, Peatfield RC, van Hille PT, et al. Thunderclap headache: is it migraine? Cephalalgia 1989;9(2):87–90.
33. Markus HS. A prospective study of thunderclap headache mimicking subarachnoid hemorrhage. J Neurol Neurosurg Psychiatry 1991;54:1117–25.
34. Linn FH, Wijdicks EF, van deer Graf Y, et al. Prospective study of sentinel headache in aneurysmal subarachnoid hemorrhage. Lancet 1994;344:590–3.
35. Landtblom AM, Fridriksson S, Boivie J, et al. Sudden onset headache: a prospective study of features, incidence and causes. Cephalalgia 2002;22:354–60.
36. Purdy RA, Kirby S. Headaches and brain tumors. Neurol Clin N Am 2004;22(1): 39–53.
37. Id Forsyth PA, Posner JB. Headaches in patients with brain tumors. Neurology 1993;43:1678–83.
38. Schankin C, Ferrari U, Reinish V, et al. Characteristics of brain tumor associated headache. Cephalalgia 2007;27(8):904–11.
39. Nahas NJ. Cluster headache and other trigeminal autonomic cephalalgias. Continuum 2021;27(3):633–51.
40. See also Levy MJ, Matharu MS, Meeran K, et al. The clinical characteristics of headache in patients with pituitary tumors. Brain 2005;128(8):1921–30.
41. Favier I, van Vliet JA, Roon KI, et al. Trigeminal autonomic cephalgias due to structural lesions. Arch Neurol 2007;64(1):25–31.

42. Johnston JC, Wester K, Sartwelle TP. Neurological fallacies leading to malpractice. Neurol Clin 2016;34:747–73.

43. Evans RW, Johnston JC. Migraine and medical malpractice. Headache 2011; 51(3):434–40.

44. Smith JH. Other primary headache disorders. Continuum 2021;27(3):652–64.

45. See also Chen PK, Fuh JL, Wang SJ. Cough headache: A study of 83 consecutive patients. Cephalalgia 2009;29(10):1079–85.

46. Pascaul J, Iglesias F, Oterino A, et al. Cough, exertional and sexual headaches. Neurology 1996;46(6):1520–4.

47. Headache Classification Committee of the International Headache Society. The international classification of headache disorders. Cephalgia 2018;38(1):1–211.

48. See generally, Aminoff MJ, Boller F Headache. Handbook of Clinical Neurology 2017, ch;97:2–825.

49. Evans RW, Burch RC, Frishberg BM, et al. Neuroimaging for Migraine: The American Headache Society Systematic Review and Evidence-Based Guideline. Headache 2020;60(2):318–36.

50. Previous iteration: United States Headache Consortium. Practice parameter: Evidence-based guidelines for migraine headache (an evidence based review): Report of the Quality Standards Subcommittee of the American Academy of Neurology. Neurology 2000;55:754–62.

51. Supra notes 42, 43. See also Hawasli AH, Chicoine MR, Dacey RG. Choosing wisely: a neurosurgical perspective on neuroimaging for headaches. Neurosurg 2015;76:1–6.

52. Supra notes 16, 42.

53. Available at: https://www.cdc.gov/stroke/facts.htm. (Accessed 10 January 2023).

54. Powers WJ, Rabinstein AA, Ackerson T, et al. Guidelines for the early management of patients with acute ischemic stroke: 2019 update to the 2018 Guidelines for the early management of acute ischemic stroke: a guideline for healthcare professionals from the American Heart Association/American Stroke Association. Stroke 2019;50:e344–418.

55. See Rabinstein AA. Update of treatment of acute ischemic stroke. Continuum (Minneap. Minn) 2020;26(2):268–86.

56. Tissue plasminogen activator for acute ischemic stroke. The National Institute of Neurological Disorders and Stroke rt-PA Stroke Study Group. N Engl J Med 1995;333:1581–7.

57. Hacke W, Kaste M, Fieschi C, et al. Intravenous thrombolysis with recombinant tissue plasminogen activator for acute hemispheric stroke: the European Cooperative Acute Stroke Study (ECASS). JAMA 1995;274:1017–25.

58. Hacke W, Kaste M, Fieschi C, et al. Randomized double-blind placebo-controlled trial of thrombolytic therapy with intravenous altepase in acute ischemic stroke (ECASS II). Lancet 1998;352:1245–51.

59. Wardlaw JM, Murray V, Berge E, et al. Thrombolysis for acute ischemic stroke. Cochrane Database Syst Rev 2014;7:CD000213.

60. Hacke W, Donnan G, Fieschi C, et al. Association of outcome with early stroke treatment: pooled analysis of ATLANTIS, ECASS, and NINDS rt-PA stroke trials. Lancet 2004;363:768–74.

61. American College of Emergency Physicians and the American Academy of Neurology. Clinical policy: use of intravenous tPA for the management of acute ischemic stroke in the emergency department. Ann Emerg Med 2013;61: 225–43.

62. Hacke W, Kaste M, Bluhmki E, et al. Thrombolysis with alteplase 3 to 4.5 hours after acute ischemic stroke. N Engl J Med 2008;359:1317–29.

63. See Jauch EC, Saver JL, Adams HP, et al. Guidelines for the early management of patients with acute ischemic stroke: a guideline for healthcare professionals from the American Heart Association/American Stroke Association. Stroke 2013; 44(3):870–947.

64. Powers WJ, Derdeyn CP, Biller J, et al. on behalf of the American Heart Association Stroke Council. 2015 American Heart Association/American Stroke Association focused update of the 2013 Guidelines for the Early Management of Patients with Acute Ischemic Stroke Regarding Endovascular Treatment. Stroke 2015;46:3020–35.

65. Kobeissi H, Ghozy S, Turfe B, et al. Tenecteplase vs alteplase for treatment of acute ischemic stroke: a systematic review and meta-analysis of randomized trials. Front Neurol 2023;14. https://doi.org/10.3389/fneur.2023.1102463.

66. MacGrory B, Saldanha IJ, Mistry EA, et al. Thrombolytic therapy for wake-up stroke: a systematic review and meta-analysis. Eur J Neurol 2021;28(6): 2006–16.

67. See Canterbury v. Spence, 464 F.2d 772 (D.C. Cir. 1972), cert. denied, 408 U.S. 1064 (1974) and its progeny.

68. Kass JS, Rose RV. Legal liability associated with rtPA administration and surrogate decision makers. Continuum 2020;26(2):499–505.

69. See also Silva GS, Nogueira RG. Endovascular treatment of acute ischemic stroke. Continuum 2020;26(2):310–31.

70. Nogueira RG, Jadhav AP, Haussen DC, et al. Thrombectomy 6 to 24 hours after stroke with a mismatch between deficit and infarct. N Engl J Med 2018;378(1): 11–21.

71. Albers GW, Marks MP, Kemp S, et al. Thrombectomy for stroke 6 to 16 hours with selection by perfusion imaging. N Engl J Med 2018;378(8):708–18.

72. See generally Kim AS. Medical management for secondary stroke prevention. Continuum 2020;26(2):435–56.

73. Ruff IM, Jendal JA. Use of heparin in acute ischemic stroke: is there still a role? Curr Atheroscler Rep 2015;17(9):51.

74. Supra notes 72, 73. See also Schwartz NE, Diener H, Albers GW. Antithrombotic agents for stroke prevention. In: Fisher M, editor. Stroke III: investigation and management (handbook of clinical neurology. Series 3), 94. Amsterdam, Netherlands: Elsevier; 2009. p. 1277–94 (providing a historical perspective).

75. Id. See also Go AS, Mozaffarian D, Roger VL, et al. Heart disease and stroke statistics – 2013 update: a report from the American Heart Association. Circulation 2013;127(1):e6–245.

76. Culebras A, Messe SR, Chaturvedi S, et al. Summary of evidence-based guideline update: prevention of stroke in nonvalvular atrial fibrillation. Report of the guideline development subcommittee of the American Academy of Neurology. Neurology 2014;82:716–24 (Re-affirmed 22 October 2022).

77. English J, Smith W. Cardio-embolic stroke. In: Fisher M, editor. Stroke II: clinical manifestations and pathogenesis (handbook of clinical neurology. Series 3), 93. Amsterdam, Netherlands: Elsevier; 2009. p. 719–49 (providing historical discussion).

78. Supra note 72.

79. Supra note 72. See also Connolly SJ, Ezekowitz MD, Yusuf S, et al. Dabigatran versus warfarin in patients with atrial fibrillation, N Engl J Med, 361 (12), 2009, 1139–1151.

80. Diener HC, Connolly SJ, Ezekowitz MD, et al. Dabigatran compared with warfarin in patients with atrial fibrillation and previous transient ischaemic attack or stroke: a subgroup analysis of the RE-LY trial. Lancet Neurol 2010;12(9): 1157–63.

81. Hankey GJ, Patel MR, Stevens SR, et al. Rivaroxaban versus warfarin in nonvalvular atrial fibrillation. N Engl J Med 2011;365(10):883–91.

82. Easton JD, Lopes RD, Bahit MC, et al. Apixaban compared with warfarin in patients with atrial fibrillation and previous stroke or transient ischaemic attack: a subgroup analysis of the ARISTOTLE trial. Lancet Neurol 2012;11(6):503–11.

83. Granger CB, Alexander JH, McMurray JJ, et al. Apixaban versus warfarin in patients with atrial fibrillation. N Engl J Med 2011;365(11):981–92.

84. Kleindorfer DO, Towfighi A, Chaturvedi S, et al. 2021 Guideline for the prevention of stroke in patients with stroke and transient ischemic attack. Stroke 2021;52:e364–467.

85. Id. See Brown DL, Levine DA, et al. Benefits and risks of dual versus single antiplatelet therapy for secondary stroke prevention: a systematic review for the 2021 guideline for the prevention of stroke in patients with stroke and transient ischemic attack. Stroke 2021;52:e468–79.

86. See also, Turan TN, Zaidat OO, Chimowitz MI, et al. Stroke prevention in symptomatic large artery intracranial atherosclerosis practice advisory: report of the AAN Guideline Subcommittee. Neurology 2022;98(12):486–98.

87. Supra notes 84-86.

88. Waters MF. Surgical approaches to stroke risk reduction. Continuum 2020;26(2): 457–77, summarizing the North American Symptomatic Endarterectomy Trial, European Carotid Surgery Trial, Asymptomatic Carotid Surgery Trial, Carotid Revascularization Endarterectomy versus Stenting Trial, Stenting and Aggressive Medical Management for the Prevention of Recurrent Ischemic Stroke Trial.

89. AbuRahma AR, Avgerinos ED, Chang RW, et al. Society for Vascular Surgery clinical practice guidelines for management of extracranial cerebrovascular disease. J Vasc Surg 2022;75(1S):4S–22S.

90. Bonati LH, Kakkos S, Berkefeld J, et al. European Stroke Organization guideline on endarterectomy and stenting for carotid artery stenosis. Eur Stroke J 2021; 6(2):I–XLVII.

91. See also Rothwell P. Carotid endarterectomy, stenting, and other prophylactic interventions. In: Fischer M, editor. Stroke III: investigation and management (handbook of clinical neurology94. Amsterdam, Netherlands: Elsevier; 2009. p. 1295–325.

92. See also Brott TG, Halperin JL, Abbara S, et al. ASA/ACCF/AHA/AANN/AANS/ ACR/ASNR/CNS/SAIP/SCAI/SIR/SNIS/SVM/SVS Guideline on the management of patients with extracranial carotid and vertebral artery disease. Circulation 2011;124:e54–130.

93. Supra notes 88-92.

94. Supra notes 88, 89, and 92.

95. Supra notes 88, 92. See also Silver FL, Mackey A, et al. Safety of stenting and endarterectomy by symptomatic status in the Carotid Revascularization Endarterectomy Versus Stenting Trial (CREST), Stroke, 42 (3), 2011, 675–680.

96. Carotid Stenting Trialists' Collaboration, Bonati LH, Dobson J, Algra A, et al. Short-term outcome after stenting versus endarterectomy for symptomatic carotid stenosis: a preplanned meta-analysis of individual patient data. Lancet 2010;376(9746):1062–73.

97. CDC Epilepsy at. Available at: https://www.cdc.gov/epilepsy/about/fast-facts. htm. (Accessed 10 January 2023).
98. See also Epilepsy Foundation at Available at: https://www.epilepsy.com/learn/about-epilepsy-basics/epilepsy-statistics. (Accessed 10 January 2023).
99. WHO at Available at: https://www.who.int/news-room/fact-sheets/detail/epilepsy. (Accessed 10 January 2023).
100. See generally. In: Engel J, Pedley T, editors. Epilepsy: a comprehensive textbook. 2nd edition. Philadelphia: Lippincott-Raven Publishers; 2008.
101. See, Lewis SL Epilepsy. Continuum 2022;28:230–602.
102. Krumholz A, Wiebe S, Gronseth G, et al. Evidence based guideline: management of an apparent unprovoked first seizure in adults (an evidence based review): Report of the Guideline Development Subcommittee of the American Academy of Neurology and the American Epilepsy Society. Neurology 2015; 84(16):1705–30.
103. Available at: www.epilepsyfoundation.org. Accessed 10 January 2023.
104. Tarasoff v. Regents of the University of California, 551 P.32d 334 (Cal. 1976). Almost a half century after Tarasoff, and there remain vagaries on application, differing interpretations among and within the states, and variations in applying the holding to the medical profession.
105. See Neurology and Pregnancy: neuro-obstetric disorders. In: Steegers EAP, Cipolla MJ, Miller E, editors. Handbook of clinical neurology, 172. Amsterdam: Elsevier; 2020. p. 2–275.
106. See also, Bui E. Women's issues in epilepsy. Continuum 2022;28(2):399–427.
107. Supra notes 105, 106.
108. Supra note 81. See also Holmes L, Harvey E, Coull B, et al. The teratogenicity of anticonvulsant drugs. N Engl J Med 2001;344(15):1132–8, and extensive subsequent studies, reports, and registries.
109. Harden CL, Meador KJ, Pennell PB, et al. Practice parameter update: Management issues for women with epilepsy – Focus on pregnancy (an evidence based review): Teratogenesis and perinatal outcomes. Report of the Quality Standards Subcommittee and Therapeutics and Technology Assessment Subcommittee of the American Academy of Neurology and American Epilepsy Society. Neurology 2009;73:133–41. Re-affirmed 22 October 2022.
110. Id.
111. Wyszynski D, Nambisan M, Survet T, et al. Increased rate of major malformations in offspring exposed to valproate during pregnancy. Neurology 2005;64: 961–5.
112. Meador KJ, Baker GA, Browning N, et al. Cognitive function at 3 years of age after fetal exposure to antiepileptic drugs. NEJM 2009;360:1597–605.
113. Vajda FJE, O'Brien TJ, Lander CM, et al. The teratogenicity of the newer antiepileptic drugs – an update. Acta Neurol Scand 2014;130(4):234–8.
114. Hernandez-Diaz S, Smith CR, Shen A, et al. Comparative safety of antiepileptic drugs during pregnancy. Neurology 2012;78(21):1692–9.
115. Jentink J, Loane MA, Dolk H, et al. EUROCAT Antiepileptic Study Working Group. Valproic acid monotherapy in pregnancy and major congenital malformations. N Engl J Med 2010;362(23):2185–93.
116. Hunt S, Russell A, Smithson WH, et al. Topiramate in pregnancy: preliminary experience from the UK Epilepsy and Pregnancy Registry. Neurology 2008; 71(4):272–6.
117. Jentink J, Dolk H, Loane MA, et al. EUROCAT Antiepileptic Study Working Group. Intrauterine exposure to carbamazepine and specific congenital

malformations: systematic review and case-control study. BMJ 2010;341:c6581. See also, Supra notes 89 and 92.

118. See also National Birth Defects Prevention Study, Werler MM, Ahrens KA, Bosco JL, et al. Use of antiepileptic medications in pregnancy in relation to risks of birth defects. Ann Epidemiol 2011;21(11):842–50.

119. American Epilepsy Society Position Statement on the Use of Valproate by Women of Childbearing Potential. Updated 8 June 2021.

120. Margulis AV, Mitchell AA, Gilboa SM, et al. Use of topiramate in pregnancy and risk of oral clefts. Am J Obstet Gynecol 2012;207(5):405.e1–7.

121. Supra note 108.

122. Supra note 109. See also, Tomson T, Battino D, Bonizzoni E, et al. EURAP study group. Dose-dependent risk of malformations with antiepileptic drugs: an analysis of data from the EURAP epilepsy and pregnancy registry, *Lancet Neurol*, 10 (7), 2011, 609–617.

123. Harden CL, Hopp J, Ting TY. Practice parameter update: Management issues for women with epilepsy – Focus on pregnancy (an evidence based review): Obstetrical complications and change in seizure frequency. Report of the Quality Standards Subcommittee and Therapeutics and Technology Assessment Subcommittee of the American Academy of Neurology and American Epilepsy Society. Neurology 2009;73:126–32. Re-affirmed 22 October 2022.

124. Harden CL, Pennell PB, Koppel BS. Practice parameter update: Management issues for women with epilepsy – Focus on pregnancy (an evidence based review): Vitamin K, folic acid, blood levels, and breastfeeding. Report of the Quality Standards Subcommittee and Therapeutics and Technology Assessment Subcommittee of the American Academy of Neurology and American Epilepsy Society. Neurology 2009;73:142–9. Re-affirmed 22 October 2022.

125. Supra note 109.

126. Supra note 124. Czeizel A.E., Prevention of congenital abnormalities by periconceptional multivitamin supplementation, *BMJ*, 306 (6893), 1993, 1645–1648, Other studies have not demonstrated a benefit of folic acid supplementation in reducing the risk of major congenital malformations.

127. See, e.g. Morrow JI, Hunt SJ, Russell AJ, et al. Folic acid use and major congenital malformations in offspring of women with epilepsy: a prospective study from the UK Epilepsy and Pregnancy Register J Neurol Neurosurg Psychiatry 2009; 80(5):506–11. At least eight studies demonstrate that folic acid supplementation may have a beneficial effect on cognitive development

128. See, e.g. Meador KJ, Baker GA, Browning N, et al. NEAD Study Group. Fetal antiepileptic drug exposure and cognitive outcomes at age 6 years (NEAD Study): a prospective observational study Lancet Neurol 2013;12(3):244–52

129. Available at: https://www.guidelinecentral.com/guideline/308468/Cheschier N. (Accessed 12 January 2023).

Protecting Privacy

Health Insurance Portability and Accountability Act of 1996, Twenty-First Century Cures Act, and Social Media

Rachel V. Rose, JD, MBA[a,b], Abhay Kumar, MD[c],
Joseph S. Kass, MD, JD[b,d,e],*

KEYWORDS

- Privacy rule • HIPAA • Twenty-First Century Cures Act • Information blocking
- Social media

KEY POINTS

- The Health Insurance Portability and Accountability Act of 1996 (HIPAA) Privacy Rule requires patient receipt of a written notice of privacy practices, patient consent for release of most protected health information to third parties, and timely release of most types of medical records to patients.
- Information blocking is a practice that interferes with a patient's access, exchange, or use of electronic health information (EHI).
- Under both HIPAA and the Twenty-First Century Cures Act, covered entities, including neurologists, must provide certain EHI to patients without interference.
- Looking up a patient online may seem like accessing any other public information about the patient, but such activity may infringe on a patient's trust and therefore be entirely unjustifiable if performed with voyeuristic intent.
- An online search of a patient's social media may adversely impact the physician–patient relationship and yield information that cannot be acted on in a clearly defined manner.

[a] Rachel V. Rose – Attorney At Law PLLC, PO Box 22718, Houston, TX 77227, USA; [b] Center for Medical Ethics & Health Policy, Baylor College of Medicine, One Baylor Plaza, Houston, TX 77030, USA; [c] Vivian L. Smith Department of Neurosurgery, McGovern Medical School at UTHealth Houston, 6400 Fannin Street, MSB 7.154, Houston, TX 77030, USA; [d] Department of Neurology, Baylor College of Medicine, 7200 Cambridge Street 9th Floor, Houston, TX 77030, USA; [e] Menninger Deptartment of Psychiatry and Behavioral Sciences, Baylor College of Medicine, Houston, TX, USA
* Corresponding author. Department of Neurology, Baylor College of Medicine, 7200 Cambridge Street 9th Floor, Houston, TX 77030.
E-mail address: kass@bcm.edu
Twitter: @JosephKass4 (J.S.K.)

Neurol Clin 41 (2023) 513–522
https://doi.org/10.1016/j.ncl.2023.03.007
0733-8619/23/© 2023 Elsevier Inc. All rights reserved.
neurologic.theclinics.com

OVERVIEW

The legal expectation of privacy, especially in health care, is not new in American law. As early as 1891, the US Supreme Court opined that "[n]o right is held more sacred, or is more carefully guarded, by the common law, than the right of every individual to the possession and control of his own person."[1] Fast forward approximately 130 years, and this premise remains both an ethical and legal *sine qua non* of the physician–patient relationship.

> *A confidential relationship between physician and patient is essential for the free flow of information necessary for sound medical care. Only in a setting of trust can a patient share the private feelings and personal history that enable the physician to comprehend fully, diagnose logically, and treat properly.*[2]

Not surprisingly, the American Medical Association (AMA) Code of Ethics states that "[p]rotecting information gathered in association with the care of the patient is a core value in health care."[3]

Although physicians and other health care professionals are ethically and legally obligated to protect patient privacy in all its forms, private personal information gathered in the health care context, referred to in statutory language as *protected health information* (PHI),[4] has grown increasingly vulnerable to exfiltration, manipulation, and abuse.[5] Health care providers and the organizations that manage and store PHI serve on the frontline of the battle to protect PHI and must therefore remain vigilant about the legal obligations and regulatory mechanisms promoting privacy protection and legal compliance. This article aims to explain the ethical and legal landscape related to patient privacy protection with special attention to the Health Insurance Portability and Accountability Act of 1996 (HIPAA), the Twenty-First Century Cures Act, and social media use.

THE PRIVACY RULE OF THE HEALTH INSURANCE PORTABILITY AND ACCOUNTABILITY ACT OF 1996

After HIPAA was signed into law on August 21, 1996, the US Department of Health and Human Services (HHS) promulgated a series of rules such as the Privacy Rule, Security Rule, and Breach Notification Rule, which operationalized the law.[6]

> *A major goal of the Privacy Rule is to assure that individuals' health information is properly protected while allowing the flow of health information needed to provide and promote high quality health care and to protect the public's health and well being.*[7]

Violation of any one of these three rules constitutes an HIPAA violation. The Privacy Rule established the three entities that must comply with HIPAA: a *covered entity*, a *business associate*, and a *subcontractor*.[8] A *covered entity* referrals to a health plan, a health care clearing house, or a health care provider who transmits PHI in electronic form in connection with a transaction covered by the regulation.[8] A *business associate* is a person who creates, receives, maintains, or transmits PHI on behalf of a covered entity for a purpose set forth in the definition.[8] A *subcontractor* "creates, receives, maintains, or transmits [PHI] on behalf of the business associate."[8] Some states have expanded the definition of *covered entity* to include other groups not explicitly mentioned in HIPAA regulations, so health care providers and other PHI handling entities must comply with both federal and state privacy regulations.[9]

The Privacy Rule imposes a variety of obligations for *covered entities* and *business associates*.

- Covered entities are required to provide a written notice of privacy practices, which sets forth the individual's rights related to his/her PHI and the privacy practices of health care providers and health plans in basic language.[10]
- In the absence of an explicit exception, such as a statutory requirement disclosei certain diseases to a governmental public health entity, *covered entities* must obtain authorization to disclose PHI, preferably by requiring the patient or the patient's legally authorized representative to complete a written HIPAA Authorization Form.[11]
- Right of Access requires that patients be provided a copy of their designated health record set.[12] Before disclosure, the covered entity must verify that the person requesting the information is authorized to do so.[13] "For those covered entities providing individuals with access to their PHI through Web portals, those portals should already be set up with appropriate authentication controls, as required by 45 CFR 164.312(d) of the HIPAA Security Rule, to ensure that the person seeking access is the individual or the individual's personal representative."[7]
- Right of Access covers neither psychotherapy notes[14] nor information compiled in reasonable anticipation of a legal proceeding, whether civil, criminal, or administrative.[15] However, "the underlying PHI from the individual's medical or payment records or other records used to generate the above types of excluded records or information remains part of the designated record set and subject to access by the individual."[7]

HIPAA also mandates that patients be provided with timely access to their medical records, defined as within 30 days.[16] However, states often require that medical records are provided in less than 30 days. For example, the Texas Administrative Code § 165.2(b) expressly references HIPAA but requires covered entities to provide medical and billing records within 15 days.[17] Covered entities and business associates must have processes in place to provide medical and financial records to patients within the requisite timeframe while simultaneously protecting patient privacy and remaining vigilant about cybersecurity.

UNDERSTANDING THE TWENTY-FIRST CENTURY CURES ACT: PROVIDING MEDICAL RECORDS TO PATIENTS

The Twenty-First Century Cures Act of 2016 (Cures Act) addresses interoperability, information blocking, and Office of the National Coordinator (ONC)[18] Health Information Technology (IT) Certification, expands the right of patients to access their electronic health information (EHI), and requires providers to give patients access to their EHI in the form of their choosing.[19] Cures Act Section 4004 addresses "information blocking," which is germane to maintaining a secure IT environment and providing patients access to their medical records. The Cures Act, as well as the two final rules (ONC Final Rule and Center for Medicare and Medicaid Services [CMS] Final Rule[20])[21] implementing the Cures Act, is dense and has provisions whose significance is not obvious on the first read.

"Information blocking is a practice by a health IT developer of certified health IT, health information network, health information exchange, or health care provider that except as required by law or specified by HHS as a reasonable and necessary activity is likely to interfere with access, exchange, or use of EHI." As set forth in 45 C.F.R. §.171.102:

EHI means electronic PHI as defined in 45 CFR 160.103 to the extent that it would be included in a designated record set as defined in 45 CFR 164.501, regardless of whether the group of records are used or maintained by or for a covered entity as defined in 45 CFR 164.103, but EHI shall not include (1) psychotherapy notes as defined in 45 CFR 164.501 or (2) information compiled in reasonable anticipation of, or for use in, a civil, criminal, or administrative action or proceeding.[22]

Under both HIPAA and the Twenty-first Century Cures Act, covered entities, including neurologists, must provide certain EHI to patients without interference. Failure to comply may be considered information blocking.[23] Although Section 4004 of the Cures Act establishes the general prohibition against the following forms of information blocking, it also provides eight exceptions.[8] The following practices likely constitute information blocking.

- Practices that restrict authorized access, exchange, or use under applicable state or federal law of such information for treatment and other permitted purposes under such applicable law, including transitions between certified health information technologies (health ITs).
- Implementing health IT in nonstandard ways that are likely to substantially increase the complexity or burden of accessing, exchanging, or using EHI.
- Implementing health IT in ways that are likely to (a) restrict the access, exchange, or use of EHI with respect to exporting complete information sets or in transitioning between health IT systems or (b) lead to fraud, waste, or abuse, or impede innovations and advancements in health information access, exchange, and use, including care delivery enabled by health IT.

The exceptions stipulated in Section 4004 of the Cures Act's create a balance between cybersecurity considerations, a covered entity's or business associate's obligations to other patients and its overall IT security, and an individual's right to access his/her medical records in a format of his/her choosing.[24] **Table 1** sets forth the exceptions to information blocking.[25] There are two categories of exceptions related to providing patients with EHI: (1) not fulfilling requests and (2) exceptions involving the procedures for fulfilling requests.

These eight exceptions (ie, health care providers, health IT developers, health information networks, and health information exchanges) recharacterize the conduct, so it is not considered information blocking if all the requirements for the individual exception are met.

Consider a practical example: a patient requests his/her EHI from a physician's electronic health record system to be sent to their TikTok or other social media account. First, the physician's office, as a covered entity, has an obligation to provide the patient with the requested records within 30 days unless notice is given and a valid reason exists for an additional 30-day extension.[27] Second, patients generally have the right to request that their EHI be sent to the location of their choosing. Third, the fact that a location such as TikTok or some unknown app is the requested receiving point does not mean that the physician's office or its business associate must comply. Finally, the appropriate Cures Act exception must be identified, and written notice must be provided to the patient stating that the requested delivery location is not possible, state the exception that applies, and provide an alternative method/location (ie, secure email). This balances the covered entity's obligation to provide the EHI to the patient within 30 days with its parallel obligation to protect a patient's privacy and the overall cybersecurity of its IT infrastructure and electronic health records.

THE INTERSECTION OF MEDICAL ETHICS AND SOCIAL MEDIA

Social media may be defined as "forms of electronic communication (such as websites for social networking and microblogging) through which users create online

Table 1
Exceptions to information blocking

Category of the Exception	Exception
Not fulfilling requests to access, exchange, or use EHI	*Preventing Harm Exception* applies when an actor engages in practices that are reasonable and necessary to prevent harm to a patient or another person, provided certain conditions are met.
Not fulfilling requests to access, exchange, or use[1] EHI	*Privacy Exception* applies if an actor does not fulfill a request to access, exchange, or use EHI to protect an individual's privacy, provided certain conditions are met.[26]
Not fulfilling requests to access, exchange, or use EHI	*Security Exception* applies if an actor interferes with the access, exchange, or use of EHI to protect the security of EHI, provided certain conditions are met. Note that the actions must be directly related to safeguarding the confidentiality, integrity, and availability of EHI that is tailored to specific security risks and implemented in a uniform and non-discriminatory manner.
Not fulfilling requests to access, exchange, or use EHI	*Infeasibility Exception* applies if an actor does not fulfill a request to access, exchange, or use EHI due to the infeasibility of the request, provided certain conditions are met.
Not fulfilling requests to access, exchange, or use EHI	*Health IT Performance Exception* applies when an actor takes reasonable and necessary measures to make health IT temporarily unavailable or to degrade the health ITs performance for the benefit of the overall performance of the health IT; provided certain conditions are met.
Exceptions that involve procedures for fulfilling requests to access, exchange, or use EHI	*Content and Manner Exception* is available to an actor to limit the content of its response to a request to access, exchange, or use EHI or the way it fulfills a request to access, exchange, or use EHI; provided certain conditions are met.
Exceptions that involve procedures for fulfilling requests to access, exchange, or use EHI	*Fees Exception* enables an actor to charge fees, including fees that result in a reasonable profit margin, for accessing, exchanging, or using EHI, provided certain conditions are met. Note that must comply with § 170.402(a)(4) or § 170.404.
Exceptions that involve procedures for fulfilling requests to access, exchange, or use EHI	*Licensing Exception* allows for an actor to license interoperability elements for EHI to be accessed, exchanged, or used, provided certain conditions are met.

communities to share information, ideas, personal messages, and other content (such as videos)."[28] Since the early 2000s, several widely known social media networks have emerged and are used frequently by patients and physicians alike.[29] Nearly 65% of physicians reported having interactions on various social media platforms for professional reasons.[30] In addition to using social media as a tool for marketing their practices, networking with other health care individuals, and disseminating health information to the public, physicians have increasingly opted to interact with patients on these platforms. Using social media to interact with patients requires heightened safeguards and imposes additional responsibility for protecting the confidentiality, integrity, and availability of PHI.

Both the AMA and the American Academy of Neurology have published official guidance on the use of social media in health care, covering a range of topics including looking up a patient online, connecting with a patient through a social media platform, ensuring patient privacy and confidentiality, and maintaining patient–physician boundaries.[31,32] The principles of patient autonomy, beneficence, nonmaleficence, and justice remain steadfast guides to determining the types of social media interactions in which physicians may engage while remaining true to the ethical practice of medicine.[32] These fundamental ethical principles require physicians to respect a patient's right to self-determination and to communicate honestly with patients. Physicians must also promote patient health and welfare without causing additional harm. Physicians must remain aware of the impact of their actions on society, working to ensure that the benefits and burdens of health care are distributed fairly.

Consider some practical applications of these ethical principles to physicians' social media usage: looking up a patient online may seem like accessing any other public information about the patient, but such activity may infringe on a patient's trust and therefore be entirely unjustifiable if performed with voyeuristic intent. An online search of a patient's social media may adversely impact the physician–patient relationship and yield information that a healthcare professional cannot act on in a clearly defined manner.[33] Connecting with patients using social media may not be appropriate, especially if the physician initiates such contact. A patient may feel coerced into communicating with the physician because of the inherent power differential in patient–physician relationships. Contact initiated by patients or patients' families may be problematic too, as such communication opens up the possibility to either exchanging patient–specific health care-related information on non-HIPAA compliant platforms or engaging in social interactions that may inappropriately impact the patient–physician relationship.

Example:

1. A patient's spouse requested a LinkedIn connection with the physician who led the treatment team caring for the patient after admission for a traumatic subdural hematoma. The spouse was very appreciative of the patient's care and thanked the physician for the excellent care provided in a private message. No further contact has been made since except for a commendation on the physician's work anniversary.

   Comment: This interaction is probably appropriate, as it does not involve any exchange of PHI or patient—physician boundary violations.

2. The physician received a private message recently in which the patient's spouse mentions that since hospital discharge the patient has started experiencing headaches as well as some worrisome behavioral changes. The spouse requests recommendations on appropriate next steps.

   Comment: This conversation is likely inappropriate as the platform is not a HIPAA compliant messaging platform. The physician should call the spouse to ensure the patient is safe and provide further recommendations (eg, an expedited office visit with brain imaging) while reminding the spouse that further communication should be conducted via the hospital-provided HIPAA compliant messaging system, which protects patient privacy while documenting conversations in the patient's electronic health record.

Posting on social media should be carried out with particular attention to ethical principles and in compliance with state and federal privacy protection laws. A good rule of thumb is that health care professionals should only post material appropriate for a public venue.[31] The AMA recommends posting information that is deidentified unless explicit consent has been obtained from either the patient or the patient's legal surrogate.[30] It is not uncommon for physicians to post content that can result in a violation of patient privacy, even if unintentional.[34] Some social media platforms place the onus of obtaining consent to post content on the poster.[35] Some advocate affixing the hashtag #consentobtained to patient-related online content to indicate explicitly that consent was obtained.[36] Even when proper consent is obtained, many risks to patient privacy and confidentiality remain. Content posted on social media, even if in a closed group setting, can be used by the social media company.[35,37] This information can also be hacked from these platforms for malicious use. Of course, patients are at liberty to upload their privileged information on the social media platforms at the risk of their privacy.

Case: A professional football player suffers from a concussion during an on-field collision and requires admission to the city hospital. The team caring for him includes a neurologist who has a large social media presence on Twitter and is asked by her followers about the player's progress. The neurologist declines to respond to the individual questions and instead tells her followers to read the official communication released by the hospital. After 24 hours, the player posts details about his symptoms, his imaging findings, and his prognosis for recovery.

Comment: Here, the neurologist is striving to ensure patient privacy and confidentiality in compliance with HIPAA by declining to comment about patient specifics, even though commenting on the patient's status would have increased her online popularity. The player is entitled to release information about himself to his followers.

SUMMARY

Health care professionals have long navigated the complex web of regulations protecting PHI, yet advances in EHR technology, the ever-expanding use of social media, and cybersecurity sabotage continue to threaten patient privacy and render physicians and health care organizations liable for violating federal and state laws. Violating a patient's privacy is an ethical breach with potentially serious legal and reputational consequences. A discussion of all the financial penalties that the federal government may impose for HIPAA violations is beyond the scope of this article, but health care professionals should understand that even an unintentional HIPAA violation can result in financial penalties and reputational harm. HIPAA penalties are not, however, "one-size-fits-all" but rather consider the circumstances surrounding the privacy breach. A Tier 1 violation, where "the covered entity was unaware of and could not have realistically avoided" the violation yields the lowest penalty, whereas a Tier 4 violation, which involves "willful neglect" without an attempt to take corrective action within 30 days of the violation elicits the stiffest civil penalties.[38] Furthermore, violating HIPAA for nefarious aims may result in criminal action against the perpetrator.[38] Staying complaint with HIPAA requires vigilance on the part of both individuals with legitimate access to PHI and the organizations handling that PHI. Health care professionals who post about medical issues on social media should be particularly careful that their posts comply with privacy rules. Whereas a generic brain MRI without patient identifying information will not violate HIPAA, a unique case description traceable to a specific health care institution that allows others to identify the patient is likely to have crossed the HIPAA compliance line.

CLINICS CARE POINTS

- Health care professionals should only post material on social media appropriate for a public venue.

- The American Medical Association recommends posting information that is deidentified unless explicit consent has been obtained from either the patient or the patient's legal surrogate.

- An online search of a patient's social media may adversely impact the physician–patient relationship and yield information that cannot be acted on in a clearly defined manner.

- Connecting with patients using social media may not be appropriate, especially if the physician initiates such contact. A patient may feel coerced into communicating with the physician because of the inherent power differential in patient–physician relationships.

- Contact initiated by patients or patients' families over social media may be problematic, as such communication opens the possibility of either exchanging protected health information on non-Health Insurance Portability and Accountability Act of 1996 compliant platforms or engaging in social interactions that may impact the patient–physician relationship.

DISCLOSURE

The authors have nothing to disclose.

REFERENCES

1. Union Pac. Ry. Co. v. Botsford, 141 U.S. 250 (May 25, 1891).
2. The American Academy of Family Physicians (AAFP), Confidentiality, Patient/ Physician. Available at: https://www.aafp.org/about/policies/all/confidentiality-patient-physician.html. Accessed Jan 15, 2023.
3. AMA Principles of Medical Ethics: 3.1.1. Available at: https://code-medical-ethics.ama-assn.org/sites/default/files/2022-08/3.1.1.pdf. Accessed Jan 31, 2023.
4. 45 CFR § 160.103. means information in any form or medium that is received by Business Associate from or on behalf of Covered Entity, is created by Business Associate, or is made accessible to Business Associate by Covered Entity regarding the past, present or future physical/mental condition of an individual, the provision of health care to an individual, or the past, present or future payment for the provision of health care to an individual, and that identifies the individual or with respect to which there is a reasonable basis to believe the information can be used to identify the individual. For purposes of this article, PHI is used generally to also include electronic protected health information (ePHI) (also defined in 45 CFR §160.103), and electronic health information ("EHI") as defined in 45 CFR § 171.102.
5. U.S. Department of Justice, Former Hospital Employee Indicted for Criminal HIPAA Violations (Jul. 3, 2014). Available at: https://www.justice.gov/usao-edtx/pr/former-hospital-employee-indicted-criminal-hipaa-violations; see also CISA, Ransomware Activity Targeting Healthcare and Public Health Sector, https://www.cisa.gov/uscert/ncas/alerts/aa20-302a. (last revised Nov. 2, 2020).
6. Centers for Medicare and Medicaid Services, HIPAA Basics for Providers: Privacy, Security, & Breach Notification Rules. Available at: https://www.cms.gov/

Outreach-and-Education/Medicare-Learning-Network-MLN/MLNProducts/ Downloads/HIPAAPrivacyandSecurity.pdf. Accessed Jan. 15, 2023.

7. HHS. Summary of the HIPAA Privacy Rule. Available at: https://www.hhs.gov/ hipaa/for-professionals/privacy/laws-regulations/index.html. Accessed Jan. 21, 2023.

8. 45 CFR § 160.103. Available at: https://www.ecfr.gov/current/title-45/subtitle-A/ subchapter-C/part-160. Accessed Jan. 15, 2023.

9. Texas Health and Safety Code Section 181 (defining "the term 'covered entity' [to] include a business associate, health care payer, governmental unit, information or computer management entity, school, health researcher, health care facility, clinic, health care provider, or person who maintains an Internet site."). Available at: https://statutes.capitol.texas.gov/Docs/HS/htm/HS.181.htm.

10. HHS, Model Notices of Privacy Practices. Available at: https://www.hhs.gov/ hipaa/for-professionals/privacy/guidance/model-notices-privacy-practices/index. html. Accessed Jan. 21, 2023.

11. 45 CFR § 164.524(b)(1). Available at: https://www.ecfr.gov/current/title-45/ subtitle-A/subchapter-C/part-164.

12. 45 CFR § 164.501.

13. 45 CFR § 164.514(h).

14. 45 CFR § 164.524(a)(1)(i) and § 164.501.

15. 45 CFR § 164.524(a)(1)(ii).

16. Raths, D., OCR Announces 11 Enforcement Actions in Right of Access Initiative (July 21, 2022). Available at: https://www.hcinnovationgroup.com/cybersecurity/ hipaa/news/21274953/ocr-announces-11-enforcement-actions-in-right-of-access-initiative.

17. Texas Secretary of State. 165.2 Texas Administrative Code. Available at: https:// texreg.sos.state.tx.us/public/readtac$ext.TacPage?sl=R&app=9&p_dir=&p_rloc= &p_tloc=&p_ploc=&pg=1&p_tac=&ti=22&pt=9&ch=165&rl=2. Accessed Jan 21, 2023.

18. ONC is the Office of the National Coordinator for Health Information and is organizationally located within the U.S. Department of Health and Human Services. "ONC is the principal federal entity charged with coordination of nationwide efforts to implement and use the most advanced health information technology and the electronic exchange of health information." Available at: www.heatlhit. gov/topic. (Accessed Jan 31, 2023).

19. Pub. L. 114-255 (Dec. 13, 2016). ONC Health IT Certification was initially launched in 2010 as part of the program formerly known as the Medicare and Medicaid EHR Incentive Program and renamed the Promoting Interoperability Programs. Available at: https://www.congress.gov/114/plaws/publ255/PLAW-114publ255.pdf.

20. Information blocking is mentioned fewer than 10 times in the CMS Final Rule. Therefore, the CMS Final Rule is not a focus of this publication. Available at: https://www.healthit.gov/topic/oncs-cures-act-final-rule.

21. Rose, R.V., Two final rules related to 21st Century Cures Act released during pandemic (Apr. 23, 2020). Available at: https://www.physicianspractice.com/ view/two-final-rules-related-21st-century-cures-act-released-during-pandemic. Accessed Jan 21, 2023.

22. 45 C.F.R. § 171.102. Available at: https://www.law.cornell.edu/cfr/text/45/171.102. Accessed Jan. 21, 2023.

23. 45 C.F.R. § 171.103. Available at: https://www.law.cornell.edu/cfr/text/45/171.103. Accessed Jan. 21, 2021.

24. ONC's Cures Act Final Rule supports seamless and secure access, exchange, and use of electronic health information. Available at: https://www.healthit.gov/curesrule/(last visited May 31, 2021). See ONC, Cure Act Final Rule – Application Programming Interfaces (APIs) Conditions and Maintenance of Certification, (last visited Jan. 19, 2023) (emphasizing Section 4002 of the Cures Act and the requirements of Certification for health IT developers participating in the ONC Health IT Certification Program).

25. ONC Cures Act Final Rule Information Blocking Exceptions. Available at: https://www.healthit.gov/cures/sites/default/files/cures/2020-03/InformationBlockingExceptions.pdf. Accessed Jan. 13, 2023.

26. The HIPAA Privacy Rule, 45 C.F.R. § 164.525(a)(1), (2), applies.

27. 45 C.F.R. § 164.524; see also. Available at: https://www.hhs.gov/hipaa/for-professionals/privacy/guidance/access/index.html. Accessed Jan. 21, 2023.

28. Merriam-Webster. Social media. Available at: https://www.merriam-webster.com/dictionary/social%20media. Accessed Jan. 15, 2023.

29. K. Hines, The History of Social Media. Available at: https://www.searchenginejournal.com/social-media-history/462643/#close. Sept. 2, 2022.

30. Modahl M., Tompsett L., Moorhead T., et al., Doctors, patients, & social media, 2011, Chief Executive. Available at: https://chiefexecutive.net/.

31. American Medical Association, Professionalism in the Use of Social Media (Opinion 2.3.2). Available at: https://code-medical-ethics.ama-assn.org/ethics-opinions/professionalism-use-social-media. Accessed Jan. 15, 2023.

32. Busl KM, Rubin MA, Tolchin BD, et al. Use of social media in health care—opportunities, challenges, and ethical considerations. Neurology 2021;97(12):585. LP – 594.

33. Chretien KC, Kind T. Social media and clinical care: ethical, professional, and social implications. Circulation 2013;127(13). https://doi.org/10.1161/CIRCULATIONAHA.112.128017.

34. Hernandez JA, Glener AD, Rosenfield LK. #Trending: why patient identifying information should be protected on social media. Plast Reconstr Surg 2021;148(4):699e–700e.

35. Twitter Terms of Service. (n.d.). Available at: https://twitter.com/en/tos. Accessed January 25, 2023.

36. Kumar A, Chen N, Singh A. #ConsentObtained – Patient Privacy in the Age of Social Media. J Hosp Med 2020;15(11):702–4.

37. Facebook. (n.d.). Available at: https://www.facebook.com/terms.php;. Accessed January 25, 2023.

38. What are the Penalties for HIPAA Violations? HIPAA Journal posted January 1, 2023. Available at: https://www.hipaajournal.com/what-are-the-penalties-for-hipaa-violations-7096. Accessed February 8, 2023.

False Claims Act and Anti-Kickback Statute

Avoiding Legal Landmines

Rachel V. Rose, JD, MBA[a,b], Joseph S. Kass, MD, JD[c,d,e],*

KEYWORDS

- False claims act ● Anti-Kickback Statute ● Fraud ● False claims ● Cybersecurity

KEY POINTS

- The False Claims Act (FCA) prohibits submitting or causing others to submit fraudulent claims or payment requests to the federal government.
- The Anti-Kickback Statute (AKS) prohibits medical providers from receiving remuneration for referrals or the use of services or products of federal program beneficiaries with certain safe harbor exceptions.
- AKS violations also constitute FCA violations, and compliance with AKS is a condition of payment for services covered by federal programs (such as Medicaid, Medicare, and Tricare).
- The FCA is also used to enforce compliance with electronic health record cybersecurity requirements required to be in place to combat threats to the security of sensitive information and critical systems.

OVERVIEW

Medicare and Medicaid federal fraud and abuse laws include the False Claims Act (FCA); Anti-Kickback Statute (AKS); Physician Self-Referral Law (Stark Law); Social Security Act, which includes the Exclusion Statute and Civil Monetary Penalties Law; and US Criminal Code.[1] Two of these laws, the FCA and AKS, are the focus of this article because kickbacks and false claims are often brought together.

[a] Rachel V. Rose – Attorney At Law PLLC, PO Box 22718, Houston, TX 77227, USA; [b] Center for Medical Ethics & Health Policy, Baylor College of Medicine, Houston, TX, USA; [c] Department of Neurology, Baylor College of Medicine, 7200 Cambridge Street 9th Floor, Houston, TX 77030, USA; [d] Center for Medical Ethics & Health Policy; [e] Menninger Department of Psychiatry & Behavioral Sciences all at Baylor College of Medicine

* Corresponding author. Department of Neurology, Baylor College of Medicine, 7200 Cambridge Street 9th Floor, Houston, TX 77030.

E-mail address: kass@bcm.edu

Twitter: @JosephKass4 (J.S.K.)

Neurol Clin 41 (2023) 523–531
https://doi.org/10.1016/j.ncl.2023.03.006
0733-8619/23/© 2023 Elsevier Inc. All rights reserved.

neurologic.theclinics.com

Originally enacted in 1863 in response to contractor fraud during the Civil War and subsequently amended, the FCA provides "that any person who knowingly submitted false claims to the government is liable for … treble damages plus a penalty that is linked to inflation."[2] The United States may pursue an FCA violation on its own, or private citizens represented by counsel may file suit on behalf of the government against persons who have allegedly defrauded the United States.[3] The FCAs fundamental premise is that a knowing submission of a fraudulent claim to the government is unlawful. Therefore, "[t]he primary purpose of the FCA is to indemnify the government—through its restitutionary penalty provisions—against losses caused by a defendant's fraud."[4]

The FCA prohibits the following: knowingly presenting (or causing to be presented) to the federal government a false or fraudulent claim for payment or approval; knowingly making or using (or causing to be made or used) a false record or statement material to false or fraudulent claim; conspiring to commit a violation of the FCA; and knowingly concealing or knowingly and improperly avoiding or decreasing an obligation to pay or transmit money to the government.[5]

Although some FCA actions involve claims submitted to the government that are false or fraudulent on their face, such as the submission of claims for services not rendered, the FCA's reach is not limited to these claims. "[A]ccurate claims submitted for services actually rendered may still be considered fraudulent and give rise to FCA liability if the services were rendered in violation of other laws."[6] Claims for payment submitted to any federal health care programs in violation of the AKS are false claims for purposes of the FCA.[7]

As the Third Circuit Court of Appeals stated, "The FCA's 'chief purpose… is to prevent the commission of fraud against the federal government and to provide for the restitution of money that was taken from the federal government by fraudulent means.'"[8] In fiscal year (FY) 2022, FCA settlements and judgments exceeded $2.2 billion for the fiscal year ending September 30, 2022. Collectively, the federal "government and whistleblowers were party to 351 settlements and judgments, the second-highest number of settlements and judgments in a single year."[9] These recoveries reflected recoveries under the FCA due to the payment of kickbacks in violation of the federal AKS and Stark Law as well as the U.S. Department of Justice (DOJs) new enforcement priorities—pandemic relief and cybersecurity requirements in government contracts and grants.[9]

ANTI-KICKBACK STATUE VIOLATIONS

The AKS, which has been in force for over 50 years,[10] is a statute with the potential for both criminal and civil penalties.[11] The AKS applies to all medical providers and prohibits remuneration in either cash or kind in exchange for either referrals or the use of services or products (eg, durable medical equipment, pharmaceuticals, medical devices) of government program beneficiaries (ie, Medicare, Medicaid, Tricare). The AKS has safe harbors.[12] The most recent modifications to the AKS safe harbors were published in the *Federal Register* on December 2, 2020 with most provisions becoming effective on January 19, 2021.[13]

As codified in the Patient Protection and Affordable Care Act of 2010 ("PPACA"), "a claim that includes items or services resulting from a violation of this section constitutes a false or fraudulent claim for purposes of [the FCA]."[14] According to the legislative history of the PPACA, this amendment to the AKS was intended to clarify "that all claims resulting from illegal kickbacks are considered false claims for the purpose of civil actions under the FCA, even when the claims are not submitted directly by the wrongdoers themselves."[15] Compliance with the AKS (42 U.S.C. § 1320a-7b(b)) is a condition of payment under all federal health care programs. Claims for products or services arising from kickbacks misrepresent compliance with a material condition of payment—compliance with the AKS. Specific guilty intent is not required to establish a violation of the AKS. "With respect to violations of this section, a person need not have actual knowledge of this section or specific intent to commit a violation of this section."[16]

Examples of recent cases involving kickback violations unrelated to electronic health records (EHRs) or cybersecurity include the following.

- *Biogen, Inc (Biogen)*: On September 26, 2022, the U.S. Department of Justice (DOJ) announced that Biogen agreed to pay $900 million to resolve allegations of AKS violations, which led to the submission of false and fraudulent claims to Medicare and Medicaid. In a case in which the DOJ initially declined to intervene, the whistleblower's attorneys took the pharmaceutical company to trial because it allegedly paid kickbacks to physicians in exchange for the prescription of Biogen's drugs.[17] "According to [Relator Michael Bawduniak's] complaint, from Jan. 1, 2009, through March 18, 2014, Biogen offered and paid remuneration, including in the form of speaker honoraria, speaker training fees, consulting fees and meals, to health care professionals who spoke at or attended Biogen's speaker programs, speaker training meetings or consultant programs to induce them to prescribe the drugs Avonex, Tysabri and Tecfidera, in violation of the Anti-Kickback Statute."[18]

- *Philips RS North America f/k/a Respironics, Inc (Respironics)*: On September 1, 2022, the DOJ announced that durable medical equipment (DME) manufacturer Respironics settled allegations of AKS and FCA violations for paying kickbacks to DME suppliers in the amount of nearly $24 million.[19] The government programs which were impacted include Medicare, Medicaid, and Tricare. "The settlement resolves allegations that Respironics caused DME suppliers to submit claims for ventilators, oxygen concentrators, continuous positive airway pressure (CPAP), bilevel positive airway pressure (BiPAP) machines, and other respiratory-related medical equipment that were false because Respironics provided illegal inducements to the DME suppliers. Respironics allegedly gave the DME suppliers physician prescribing data free of charge that could assist their marketing efforts to physicians."[19] In addition, Respironics entered into a separate Corporate Integrity Agreement with U.S. Department of Health and Human Services - Office of the Inspector General (HHS-OIG) lasting 5 years that requires the implementation and monitoring of a more robust compliance program.[19]

- *Kaleo Inc (Kaleo)*: On November 21, 2021, Kaleo agreed to pay $12.7 million to resolve allegations that the company caused the submission of false and fraudulent claims related to its drug Evzio—an injectable drug indicated for reversing opioid overdoses.[20] Between March 14, 2017 and April 30, 2020, Kaleo "directed prescribing doctors to send Evzio prescriptions to certain preferred pharmacies that in turn (1) submitted false prior authorization requests for Evzio that misrepresented to insurers that the prescribing physicians submitted the request when the pharmacies did so and/or contained false or misleading assertions about the patients' medical histories, such as false statements that patients had previously tried and failed less costly alternatives to Evzio and (2) dispensed Evzio without collecting or attempting to collect co-payment obligations from government beneficiaries. The United States contend[ed] that Kaleo knew of or deliberately ignored this pharmacy misconduct, but nevertheless kept directing business to these pharmacies."[21] In addition, the DOJ alleged that illegal remuneration was provided to prescribing physicians in the form of gifts. A former employee brought the case forward as a whistleblower, and she received $2,548,600 as per the FCA provision enabling a whistleblower (known as a relator in the statute) to recover a percentage of the government's recovery.[20]

- *Metric Lab Services, LLC (Metric)*: On July 22, 2022, the DOJ announced that Metric and Spectrum Diagnostic Labs LLC, as well as two individuals, agreed to pay $5.7 million to settle allegations that false and fraudulent claims were submitted to Medicare by paying kickbacks in the form of sham agreements with marketers to provide various consulting, marketing, and other services.[22] "In reality, however, Metric and Spectrum paid the marketers a percentage of revenue, including Medicare reimbursement, in return for samples. The marketers then generated sham invoices for hourly services that matched the agreed-upon kickback amount."[23] This case is notable because the two individuals had previously pled guilty to a single count of conspiracy to defraud the United States in connection with the AKS scheme.[24]
- *Arthrex, Inc (Arthrex)*: On November 8, 2021, the DOJ announced that the orthopedic medical device company Arthrex agreed to pay $16 million to resolve allegations that it caused FCA violations to Medicare from August 2010 to March 5, 2021 by paying kickbacks to an orthopedic surgeon based in Colorado.[25] "The settlement resolves allegations that Arthrex agreed to provide remuneration to the surgeon in the form of royalty payments purportedly for the surgeon's contributions to Arthrex's SutureBridge and SpeedBridge products when the remuneration was in fact intended to induce the surgeon's use and recommendation of Arthrex's products."[25]- The company also entered into a 5year Corporate Integrity Agreement with HHS-OIG.[26]

These cases demonstrate that the federal government often deploys AKS in conjunction with the FCA in cases where false and fraudulent claims are submitted to federal government programs. Reading nearly any DOJ press release related to the AKS and FCA reveals that the government and relators (aka whistleblowers) are concerned about the following three items: (1) combatting health care fraud; (2) corrupting health care professionals' independent medical decision-making; and (3) kickbacks, which "have no place anywhere in our health care system."[25] In sum, paying remuneration, in either cash or kind, whether directly or indirectly, risks both criminal and civil liability.

CYBERSECURITY AND ELECTRONIC HEALTH RECORD VIOLATIONS

In October 2021, the DOJ announced its Civil Cyber-Fraud Initiative, enabling it to use the FCA to tackle "new and emerging cyber threats to the security of sensitive information and critical systems."[27] The focus of the initiative includes the following.

- building broad resiliency against cybersecurity intrusions across the government, the public sector, and key industry partners
- holding contractors and grantees to their commitments to protect government information and infrastructure
- supporting government experts' efforts to timely identify, create, and publicize patches for vulnerabilities in commonly used information technology products and services
- ensuring that companies following the rules and investing in meeting cybersecurity requirements are not at a competitive disadvantage
- reimbursing the government and the taxpayers for the losses incurred when companies fail to satisfy their cybersecurity obligations

- improving overall cybersecurity practices that will benefit the government, private users, and the American public.[27]

In March 2022, the DOJ announced its first civil cyber-fraud settlement against Comprehensive Health Services, LLC.[28] In the interest of full disclosure, Rachel V Rose, Esq, was one of the attorneys who represented Relator Shawn Lawler, the individual who raised the cybersecurity concerns and allegations related to the company's failure to disclose to the government that patient medical records were not consistently stored on a secure EHR system and to implement the requisite technical, administrative, and physical safeguards required by the Health Insurance Portability and Accountability Act of 1996 and the related Security Rule[29] as well as the government contract provisions.

A related focus of the DOJ is EHR violations of its "Promoting Interoperability" program, formerly known as the "Meaningful Use" program. This program stems from the 2009 Health Information Technology for Economic and Clinical Health Act (HITECH Act)[30] and the 2016 Twenty-First Century Cures Act.[31] These two complementary laws require that EHR vendors wishing to obtain certification attest to the fact that their software meets U.S. Department of Health and Human Services (HHS)-mandated technical safeguards, allows patient access to digital health information, and prohibits information blocking.[32] Health care institutions are not immune either, as made plain in the 2019 FCA case, *United States ex rel.Awad v. Coffey Health System*[37], Case No. 2:16-cv-03034 (D. Kan.), whereby the hospital allegedly "falsely attested that it conducted and/or reviewed security risk analyses in accordance with requirements under a federal incentive program for the reporting periods of 2012 and 2013."[33] Since 2017, the federal government has settled seven FCA cases involving EHR vendors[34] for violations of the Meaningful Use/Interoperability Program, some of which also include AKS violations. Four of these cases were filed in the US District Court for the District of Vermont, including a recent settlement with Modernizing Medicine, Inc (ModMed), which was announced on November 1, 2022.[35] In this case, the DOJ claimed that the company conspired with Miraca, a laboratory services company, to prioritize Miraca laboratory orders and that ModMed donated its EHR to health care providers to increase laboratory orders to Miraca.[36] This lawsuit came on the heels of a January 2019 lawsuit in which Miraca, now called Inform Diagnostics, "paid $63.5 million to resolve allegations that it had violated the AKS and the Stark Law by providing to referring physicians subsidies for EHR systems and free or discounted technology consulting services."[36]

SUMMARY

Health care entities doing business with the federal government may run afoul of the FCA and AKS not only when they directly submit fraudulent claims for government reimbursement but also when they create schemes that manipulate others into submitting (whether knowingly or unknowingly) illegal claims. Manipulating the independent judgment of health care professionals financially, distorting the marketplace to provide financial gain for a particular entity at the government's expense, or rewarding health care providers (whether individuals or corporate) for either making specific referrals or using particular health care resources are all behaviors that may run afoul of both the FCA and AKS unless these arrangements are protected by a safe harbor exception. In recent years, the Department of Justice has been deploying these statutes to ensure that EHRs are built and maintained with appropriate cybersecurity protections.

CLINICS CARE POINTS

- Only bill for services performed. Both under-coding and over-coding violate the False Claims Act (FCA).
- Monetary or in-kind inducements for referring patients covered by federal programs such as Medicaid, Medicare, or Tricare, among others, for a range of goods and services, including medical services, durable medical equipment, pharmaceuticals, laboratory testing, or radiology services may violate the AKS and FCA.
- Failure to maintain an electronic health record system that complies with federally mandated cybersecurity rules violates several federal laws, including the FCA.
- Violating either the FCA or the AKS may lead to serious civil or criminal penalties.

DISCLOSURE

The authors have nothing to disclose.

REFERENCES

1. CMS. Medicare Fraud & Abuse: Prevent, Detect, Report.; 2019. Available at: https://www.cms.gov/Outreach-and-Education/Medicare-Learning-Network-MLN/MLNProducts/Downloads/Fraud-Abuse-MLN4649244.pdf. Accessed January 24, 2023.
2. U.S. Department of Justice, The False Claims Act. Available at: https://www.justice.gov/civil/false-claims-act. updated Feb. 2, 2022. Accessed January 24, 2023.
3. 31 USC 3729: False claims. Available at: https://uscode.house.gov/view.xhtml?req=granuleid:USC-prelim-title31-section3729&num=0&edition=prelim. Accessed January 24, 2023.
4. *U.S. ex rel. Schumann v. Astrazeneca Pharm., L.P.*, 769 F.3d 837, 840 (3d Cir. 2014).
5. 31 U.S.C. §§ 3729(a)(1)(A), (B), (C) and (G). Available at: https://uscode.house.gov/view.xhtml?req=granuleid:USC-prelim-title31-section3729&num=0&edition=prelim. Accessed January 24, 2023.
6. United States ex rel. Parikh v. Citizens Med. Ctr., 977 F. Supp. 2d 654, 662 (S.D. Tex. 2013) (Costa, J.), aff'd sub nom. United States ex rel. Parikh v. Brown, 762 F.3d 461 (5th Cir. 2014), opinion withdrawn and superseded on reh'g and aff'd sub nom. *United States ex rel. Parikh v. Brown,* 587 F. App'x 123 (5th Cir. 2014).
7. *United States ex rel. Thompson v. Columbia/HCA Healthcare Corp.*, 125 F.3d 899, 901-902 (5th Cir. 1997); see also *United States ex rel. King* v. Solvay, S.A., 823 F. Supp. 2d 472, 506 (S.D. Tex. 2011).
8. *U.S. ex rel. Wilkins v. United Health Grp., Inc.*, 659 F.3d 295, 304 (3d Cir. 2011) (citing *Tyson v. Wells Fargo Bank & Co.*, 78 F. Supp. 3d 360, 362 (D.D.C. 2015).
9. U.S. Department of Justice, False Claims Act Settlements and Judgments Exceed $2 Billion in Fiscal Year 2022 (Feb. 7, 2023). Available at: https://www.justice.gov/opa/pr/false-claims-act-settlements-and-judgments-exceed-2-billion-fiscal-year-2022. Accessed January 24, 2023.
10. Social Security Amendments of 1972, Pub. L. No. 92-603, §§ 242(b) and (c); 42 U.S.C. § 1320a-7b, Medicare-Medicaid Antifraud and Abuse Amendments, Pub. L. No. 95-142; Medicare and Medicaid Patient Program Protection Act of

1987, Pub. L. No. 100-93. Available at: https://www.govinfo.gov/content/pkg/STATUTE-86/pdf/STATUTE-86-Pg1329.pdf. Accessed January 24, 2023.

11. 42 U.S. Code § 1320a–7b - Criminal penalties for acts involving Federal health care programs. Available at: https://www.govinfo.gov/app/details/USCODE-2010-title42/USCODE-2010-title42-chap7-subchapXI-partA-sec1320a-7b. Accessed January 24, 2023.

12. 42 C.F.R. § 1001.952 (indicating that although certain payment and business arrangements may implicate the AKS, so long as the requirements of a safe harbor are met, the U.S. Department of Health and Human Services – Office of the Inspector General will not treat the conduct as actionable offenses under the AKS). Available at: https://www.ecfr.gov/current/title-42/chapter-V/subchapter-B/part-1001/subpart-C/section-1001.952. Accessed January 24, 2023.

13. 85 Fed. Reg. 77895 (Dec. 2, 2020). Available at: https://www.federalregister.gov/documents/2020/12/02/2020-26072/medicare-and-state-health-care-programs-fraud-and-abuse-revisions-to-safe-harbors-under-the. Accessed January 24, 2023.

14. Pub. L. No. 111-148, § 6402(f), 124 Stat. 119, codified at 42 U.S.C. § 1320a-7b(g). Available at: https://www.congress.gov/111/plaws/publ148/PLAW-111publ148.pdf. Accessed January 24, 2023.

15. 155 Cong. Rec. S10854. Statements on Introduced Bills and Joint Resolutions. Available at: https://www.govinfo.gov/app/details/CREC-2009-10-28/CREC-2009-10-28-pt1-PgS10852. Accessed January 24, 2023.

16. 42 U.S.C. § 1320a-7b(h). Criminal penalties for acts involving Federal health care programs. Available at: https://www.govinfo.gov/app/details/USCODE-2010-title42/USCODE-2010-title42-chap7-subchapXI-partA-sec1320a-7b. Accessed January 24, 2023.

17. Department of Justice. Biogen Inc. Agrees to Pay $900 Million to Settle Allegations Related to Improper Physician Payments (Sept. 26, 2022). Available at: https://www.justice.gov/opa/pr/biogen-inc-agrees-pay-900-million-settle-allegations-related-improper-physician-payments#:~:text=Biogen%20Inc.,Payments%20%7C%20OPA%20%7C%20Department%20of%20Justice. Accessed January 24, 2023.

18. Department of Justice. *United States ex rel. Bawduniak v. Biogen Idec, Inc.*, Case No. 12-cv-10601 (D. Mass.). Available at: https://www.justice.gov/d9/press-releases/attachments/2022/09/26/u.s._ex_rel._bawduniak_v._biogen_-_stipulation_of_settlement_0.pdf. Accessed January 24, 2023.

19. Department of Justice. Philips Subsidiary to Pay Over $24 Million for Alleged False Claims Caused by Respironics for Respiratory-Related Medical Equipment (Sept. 1, 2022). Available at: https://www.justice.gov/opa/pr/philips-subsidiary-pay-over-24-million-alleged-false-claims-caused-respironics-respiratory. Accessed January 24, 2023.

20. Department of Justice. Kaleo Inc. Agrees to Pay $12.7 Million to Resolve Allegations of False Claims for Anti-Overdose Drug (Nov. 9, 2021). Available at: https://www.justice.gov/opa/pr/kal-o-inc-agrees-pay-127-million-resolve-allegations-false-claims-anti-overdose-drug; see also United States ex rel. Socol v. Kaleo, Inc., Case No. 18-cv-10050 D. Mass. Accessed January 24, 2023.

21. Department of Justice. Kaleo Inc. Agrees to Pay $12.7 Million to Resolve Allegations of False Claims for Anti-Overdose Drug (Nov. 9, 2021). Available at: https://www.justice.gov/opa/pr/kal-o-inc-agrees-pay-127-million-resolve-allegations-false-claims-anti-overdose-drug; see also United States ex rel. Socol v. Kaleo, Inc., Case No. 18-cv-10050 (D. Mass.). Accessed January 24, 2023.

22. Department of Justice. Metric Lab Services, Metric Management Services LLC, Spectrum Diagnostic Labs LLC, and Owners Agree to Pay $5.7 Million to Settle Allegations of False Claims for Unnecessary Genetic Testing (Jul. 22, 2022). Available at: https://www.justice.gov/opa/pr/metric-lab-services-metric-management-services-llc-spectrum-diagnostic-labs-llc-and-owners. Accessed January 24, 2023.

23. Department of Justice. Metric Lab Services, Metric Management Services LLC, Spectrum Diagnostic Labs LLC, and Owners Agree to Pay $5.7 Million to Settle Allegations of False Claims for Unnecessary Genetic Testing (Jul. 22, 2022). Available at: https://www.justice.gov/opa/pr/metric-lab-services-metric-management-services-llc-spectrum-diagnostic-labs-llc-and-owners. Accessed January 24, 2023.

24. United States v. Kennerson, Case No. 20-cr-00448 (D.N.J.); *United States v. Madison,* Case No. 20-cr-00449 (D.N.J.).

25. Department of Justice. Medical Device Company Arthrex to Pay $16 Million to Resolve Kickback Allegations (Nov. 8, 2021). Available at: https://www.justice.gov/opa/pr/medical-device-company-arthrex-pay-16-million-resolve-kickback-allegations; see also *United States ex rel. Shea v. Arthrex Inc. et al.* Case No. 20-cv-10201 (D. Mass.). Accessed January 24, 2023.

26. Settlement Agreement (Nov. 8, 2021). Available at: https://www.justice.gov/opa/press-release/file/1447156/download. Accessed January 24, 2023.

27. Department of Justice. Deputy Attorney General Lisa O. Monaco Announces New Civil Cyber-Fraud Initiative (Oct. 6, 2021). Available at: https://www.justice.gov/opa/pr/deputy-attorney-general-lisa-o-monaco-announces-new-civil-cyber-fraud-initiative. Accessed January 24, 2023.

28. Department of Justice. Medical Services Contractor Pays $930,000 to Settle False Claims Act Allegations Relating to Medical Services Contracts at State Department and Air Force Facilities in Iraq and Afghanistan – First Settlement by the Department of Justice of a Civil Cyber-Fraud Case Under the Department's Civil Cyber-Fraud Initiative (Mar. 8, 2022). Available at: https://www.justice.gov/opa/pr/medical-services-contractor-pays-930000-settle-false-claims-act-allegations-relating-medical. Accessed January 24, 2023.

29. R. V. Rose, Cybersecurity: Look to where you are going (Feb. 11, 2021). Available at: https://www.physicianspractice.com/view/cybersecurity-look-to-where-you-are-going. Accessed January 24, 2023.

30. Pub. L. 111-5 (Feb. 17, 2009). American Recovery and Reinvestment Act of 2009. Available at: https://www.govinfo.gov/content/pkg/PLAW-111publ5/pdf/PLAW-111publ5.pdf. Accessed January 24, 2023.

31. Pub. L. 114-255 (Dec. 13, 2016). 21st Century Cures Act. Available at: https://www.govinfo.gov/content/pkg/PLAW-114publ255/pdf/PLAW-114publ255.pdf. Accessed January 24, 2023.

32. R.V. Rose, The Role of Information Blocking in Providing Patients Their Medical Records, ABA Health Law Section (Aug. 30, 2021). Available at: https://www.americanbar.org/groups/health_law/publications/health_lawyer_home/2021-august/rol-inf/. Accessed January 24, 2023.

33. Department of Justice. Kansas Hospital Agrees to Pay $250,000 To Settle False Claims Act Allegations (May 31, 2019). Available at: https://www.justice.gov/usao-ks/pr/kansas-hospital-agrees-pay-250000-settle-false-claims-act-allegations. Accessed January 24, 2023.

34. C. Matzzie, Electronic Health Records Ongoing Focus Of DOJ And HHS Enforcement (Feb. 2, 2023). https://www.taf.org/electronic-health-records-ongoing-focus-of-doj-and-hhs-enforcement/?link_id=2&can_id=d9617c866ce641a8fdf8049d4fd80783

&source=email-fraud-in-america-how-whistleblowers-exposed-the-fraud-of-trevor-milton-nikolas-founder&email_referrer=email_1806013___from_2307539&email_subject= watchdog-identifies-5-billion-in-potential-covid-aid-fraud. Accessed January 24, 2023.

35. Department of Justice. Modernizing Medicine Agrees to Pay $45 Million to Resolve Allegations of Accepting and Paying Illegal Kickbacks and Causing False Claims (Nov. 1, 2022). Available at: https://www.justice.gov/opa/pr/modernizing-medicine-agrees-pay-45-million-resolve-allegations-accepting-and-paying-illegal. Accessed January 24, 2023.

36. Milliard M. HealthcareITNews. Modernizing Medicine to pay $45M to resolve False Claims Act allegations. Available at: https://www.healthcareitnews.com/news/modernizing-medicine-pay-45m-resolve-false-claims-act-allegations. Accessed February 14, 2023.

37. Available at: https://www.justice.gov/usao-ks/pr/kansas-hospital-agrees-pay-250000-settle-false-claims-act-allegations. Accessed January 24, 2023.

Legal and Ethical Issues in the Neurology of Reproductive Health

Susan P. Raine, MD, JD, LLM, MEd

KEYWORDS

- Teratogen • Teratogenicity • Medical ethics • Neurology • Reproduction
- Shared decision-making • Epilepsy • Pregnancy

KEY POINTS

- The potential for future pregnancy in women of reproductive age impacts treatment considerations for common neurologic conditions involving potentially teratogenic medications.
- Applying ethical principles to the care and treatment of reproductive-age women emphasizes the need to weigh the risks and benefits of drug therapy in a shared decision-making model.
- Clinicians meet the legal standard of care when choosing appropriate treatment options, providing detailed counseling to the patient, consulting other specialists as needed, and documenting all aspects of care.

INTRODUCTION

Providing medical care for women who are either pregnant or may become pregnant presents unique challenges for the clinician. Chronic disease and its treatment impacts both the woman and the fetus. Typically, the interests of the mother and fetus are aligned; however, when the interests of the mother and fetus are in conflict, clinical care becomes more complex. Determining whose interests predominate can be difficult and is the subject of ethical debate, legislative action, and judicial review.

Clinical decision-making where the potential for pregnancy exists is no less complicated and is arguably even more challenging in the absence of a fetus. When pregnant, the woman presents both herself and her fetus for care with treatment decisions made based on known risks and benefits for both. When the patient is a non-pregnant woman of reproductive age, she and her physician must make medical decisions based not only on her current needs but also on the knowledge that a second patient could potentially present at any time during treatment.

Baylor College of Medicine, One Baylor Plaza, Suite N104, Houston, TX 77030, USA

Neurol Clin 41 (2023) 533–541
https://doi.org/10.1016/j.ncl.2023.03.003
0733-8619/23/© 2023 Elsevier Inc. All rights reserved.

neurologic.theclinics.com

Women are of reproductive age from menarche to menopause. The average age of menarche in the United States is between 12 and 13 years of age.[1] Menopause is diagnosed when menstruation has ceased for 12 months and occurs at a median age of 51.[2] Absent conditions definitively preventing pregnancy such as hysterectomy, women of reproductive age should be viewed as potentially fertile. Although long-acting reversible contraceptives such as intrauterine devices (IUDs) and implants are highly effective in pregnancy prevention with rates of unintended pregnancy as low as <1% with typical use, failure is possible and may result in pregnancy.[3]

DISCUSSION

Multiple neurologic conditions may impact women during their reproductive years including epilepsy, headache/migraines, myasthenia gravis, aneurysms, arteriovenous malformations, multiple sclerosis, and Guillain-Barre syndrome. Treatment of these chronic neurologic disorders has potential consequences for pregnancy that merit special consideration. In some cases, the condition itself may increase pregnancy complications. In others, the primary effect may be on a fetus, increasing the potential for harm whether the condition is treated or left untreated. Of primary concern is the potential impact of drug therapy on a developing fetus.

Several commonly prescribed medications for the treatment of neurologic disorders are either teratogens or potential teratogens. A teratogen is an agent, usually a drug, that causes fetal abnormalities following in utero exposure. Abnormalities may be structural, developmental, or both. Teratogenicity is determined by several factors including the timing of gestational exposure, dosage, number of medications taken, and the underlying disease necessitating treatment.[4] Over the past decade, more than 1 in 16 pregnancies likely involved exposure to a teratogenic drug.[5]

Teratogenic medications can have devastating effects on a developing fetus, highlighted by the thalidomide tragedy of the 1950s. Thalidomide, originally marketed in Europe and Australia as a non-addictive sedative, was noted to be a highly effective antiemetic.[6] The drug was widely prescribed in pregnancy for morning sickness, most frequently in the first trimester during a critical time in fetal development. By 1961, thalidomide was confirmed to cause severe birth defects, including limb deformities, congenital heart disease, and ocular and auditory abnormalities.[7] Thalidomide was never marketed in the United States; the Food and Drug Administration (FDA) withheld approval over safety concerns around potentially irreversible peripheral neuropathy in exposed patients and potential issues with use in pregnancy.[6]

The thalidomide experience ushered in a new era of drug safety. The Drug Amendments of 1962 increased the regulation of prescription drugs on the principle that no drug should be brought to market before proving that it is both safe and effective. As part of the strategy to achieve that goal, the FDA implemented and refined changes to drug labeling and risk mitigation strategies over the subsequent decades. To specifically address concerns around the use of medication in pregnancy, the FDA introduced a risk stratification labeling system in 1979 using letter categories (A, B, C, D, and X). Drugs with A or B labels were designated safe to use in pregnancy, category C drugs could not rule out risk to the fetus, and category D and X drugs were noted to carry a demonstrated risk of harm.[8]

Amid concerns that pregnancy categories lacked clarity, failed to provide meaningful clinical information, and were often misinterpreted and misused, the FDA replaced the risk stratification labeling system with the Pregnancy and Lactation Labeling Rule (PLLR) in 2014. Under the PLLR, pregnancy categories A, B, C, D, and X were removed from all drug products and replaced by narrative descriptions including (1) a summary of drug risks, (2) a discussion of supporting data, and (3) information to help clinicians with patient counseling and prescribing decisions. The descriptions are provided in three sections: pregnancy, lactation, and women and men of reproductive potential. The addition of reproductive potential to labeling allows for the inclusion of recommendations for pregnancy testing, and contraception in addition to fertility or pregnancy loss concerns.[9]

The FDA's efforts to improve drug labeling effectiveness have proceeded in conjunction with the agency's implementation of safety programs for drugs that may cause harm in pregnancy or have other significant side effects. In the early 2000s, the FDA created a framework for improved oversight of high-risk drugs called Risk Minimization Action Plans (RiskMAPs). Under the program, once the FDA identified the drug as high-risk, a RiskMAP for that product was requested from the manufacturer. The FDA provided drug manufacturers with general guidelines as to what information should be included, focusing on improved education about the drug's risks along with enhanced data safety and monitoring. Industry-developed RiskMAPs were voluntarily provided to the FDA.[10] In 2007, the FDA was given enforcement authority for the Risk Evaluation and Mitigation Strategy (REMS) programs that superseded RiskMAPs.[11] Drugs with the most rigorous REMS programs include Elements to Assure Safe Use (ETASU), requiring specific activities on the part of prescribers, patients, pharmacists, and drug distributors including registration, education, training, and laboratory testing.[12]

Isotretinoin, approved by the FDA in 1982 for the treatment of acne, is an early example of a drug with a sophisticated REMS program involving ETASU. Use of isotretinoin during pregnancy carries a 20% to 35% risk of birth defects in exposed fetuses, including craniofacial, cardiovascular, neurologic, and thymic malformations in addition to a high likelihood of impaired neurocognitive development.[13] Due to the drug's high teratogenic potential, Roche, the manufacturer of isotretinoin, introduced its iPLEDGE program in 2006. Under the iPLEDGE program, women are required to register on the website, use two forms of contraception for the duration of treatment, and undergo monthly pregnancy testing. There are currently only 60 drugs in the REMS program, and most drugs covered do not have an accompanying ETASU.[14]

CLINICAL RELEVANCE

Management of women with epilepsy during their reproductive years provides an excellent framework to discuss teratogenic drug use from both an ethical and a legal perspective. Approximately, 1.5 million women of childbearing age live with epilepsy, and 24,000 of these women give birth annually.[15] Many women of reproductive age control their epilepsy with known teratogenic medications such as valproic acid. Despite the risks, 60% of women in one study opted to continue with treatment either because pregnancy was highly unlikely or other treatment options had failed. Only 23% of the women treated with valproic acid were using effective contraception.[16]

Women with epilepsy who become pregnant are at increased risk of maternal morbidity and mortality, and babies born to these mothers are more likely to have congenital anomalies than women without epilepsy.[4] Prevention of seizures, particularly status epilepticus, is critical for both the pregnant woman and developing fetus and can be challenging due to the altered pharmacokinetics during pregnancy. Thus, the risks of treatment in pregnancy must be carefully weighed against the benefits of using potentially teratogenic medications to prevent pregnancy complications resulting from a worsening disease state.

Ideally, women will engage in effective family planning and delay pregnancy until their disease state is optimized, preferably with monotherapy and at the lowest possible dosage. Timing pregnancy allows for discussion of potential effects of medication on a developing fetus, preconception changes to drug therapy, prophylactic treatment such as folic acid supplementation, and consultation with a perinatologist, Women who are seizure-free for 9 to 12 months before pregnancy experience an 84% to 92% likelihood of remaining seizure-free throughout pregnancy.[15]

Even with planning, some women will become pregnant during times when they are sub-optimally controlled, taking multiple medications, or taking medications with a high risk of teratogenicity. Most major malformations occur between weeks 3 and 10 and before many women know they are pregnant. Women taking anti-seizure medications (ASMs) have a two- to three-fold increase in the rate of major congenital anomalies.[15] ASM polytherapy and use of valproate, phenobarbital, or phenytoin carry the highest risks.[15] A 2017 study found that almost 80% of women with epilepsy had an unplanned pregnancy.[15] When an unplanned pregnancy occurs, counseling from both a neurologist and a perinatologist is critical to assist the patient in understanding the possible implications for both the pregnancy and the developing fetus.

Some women with unplanned pregnancies may opt to terminate depending on their personal risk tolerance of possible fetal effects. Termination in the first trimester can be performed medically or surgically and is safest the earlier it is performed. Patients may opt to wait for a comprehensive review of fetal anatomy in the second trimester, generally completed between 18 and 20 weeks, to determine if any visible fetal anomalies are present; however, not all anomalies are detected by ultrasound and developmental delays may not be seen for several years after birth. Termination of pregnancy at 18 to 20 weeks is more technically challenging and carries a greater risk to the mother. Depending on state law, a woman may not have the option for termination.

APPROACH
Ethical Considerations

When considering how best to proceed when treating women with complex neurologic disorders during their reproductive years, it is helpful to evaluate therapeutic decisions using an ethical framework, such as the four principles of ethics: respect for autonomy, beneficence, nonmaleficence, and justice.[17]

Respect for patient autonomy recognizes the right of patients to make decisions about their care and treatment and is formally effectuated with informed consent. For a patient to provide informed consent, she must be able to understand the treatment options provided to her, how each of the options applies to her situation, the risks and benefits of undergoing treatment, and the risks and benefits of forgoing treatment. A patient with low health literacy may struggle to understand the impact of treatment on pregnancy and may thus have difficulty weighing the risks and benefits of a particular treatment course. To determine whether the patient appreciates the risks and benefits of treatment, it is important to engage in a robust discussion of the patient's response to the information provided. Through those conversations, the level of the patient's understanding becomes increasingly evident, and any deficits in knowledge can be addressed.

The ethical principle of beneficence encompasses the idea that the treating physician will act in the best interest of the patient while also exercising the duty of nonmaleficence, the ethical obligation to minimize harm. Ideally, the balance of beneficence and nonmaleficence results in a net benefit to the patient. Potential fetal effects may be considered as part of the overall balance of risks and benefits but should not be given equivalent weight. In many jurisdictions, a fetus might be granted rights that override the pregnant woman's autonomy with respect to medical decision-making, but until pregnancy occurs, the woman's interests predominate.

Justice, the fourth ethical principle, requires a fair and equitable distribution of health resources. Although approaches vary (distributive justice, rights-based justice, etc.), the core concept is that all patients are treated fairly in the context of health care decision-making. Ethical care of reproductive-age women necessitates that they should not be treated as though they were already pregnant.

Legal Considerations

Medical malpractice is a subset of tort law, an area of the law that serves to compensate individuals who have been injured by the negligence of others. For a physician to be found medically negligent, four conditions must be present. First, the physician must have a duty of care to the patient, established by virtue of a physician-patient relationship. Second, the physician must have breached that duty to care by not practicing within the standard of care. Third, physician's deviation from the standard of care must be the proximate cause of the harm, and fourth, the harm must result in a compensable harm for which damages can be awarded.

Breach of duty to care for a patient occurs when a physician fails to follow the standard of care. The standard of care is defined as the care a reasonably prudent physician would provide in the same or similar circumstances and is usually established through the testimony of expert witnesses. Evidence-based guidelines published by professional organizations are helpful in determining the standard of care but are not the final word on the standard of care.

To return to our example, when treating a woman of reproductive age with drugs that may result in harm to a developing fetus, the central issue becomes whether that treatment choice is considered the standard of care. For example, if a drug is contraindicated in pregnancy due to fetal risk but is the only effective treatment option for the patient, use of the drug would be considered standard of care despite the potential for harm. The standard of care is not limited to prescribing decisions and encompasses other aspects of patient care such as counseling, informed consent, and any other management necessary to ensure optimal treatment.

Managing women with epilepsy illustrates the various factors that determine the standard of care in the context of a medical malpractice action. As a starting point, the physician should be familiar with recommended treatment of the condition and relevant guidelines published by national organizations that may guide clinical decision-making. In 2021, the American Epilepsy Society updated its "Position Statement on the Use of Valproate by Women of Childbearing Potential".[18] Recommendations include avoiding valproate unless other treatments have failed to control the woman's symptoms, and if valproate use is necessary, the woman should use a reliable form of contraception. The guidelines also discuss the need for counseling about the risks and benefits of valproate use in pregnancy. Concurrent use of folic acid is also recommended. In this circumstance, the prescribing physician might opt to begin treatment of a reproductive-age woman with an ASM other than valproate while also counseling her on the importance of contraception and folic acid supplementation.

After settling on an appropriate treatment recommendation, the physician must counsel the patient about the reasons for the recommendation, the risks and benefits of both treatment and non-treatment, and other reasonable treatment alternatives. This discussion forms the core of the informed consent process. In addition to physician–patient agreement on the appropriate treatment option, to meet the standard of care, the treating physician should make recommendations on the need for family planning and timing of pregnancy, arrange for consultation with specialists, and ensure follow-up with the patient. All these management decisions and recommendations must be documented in the patient's medical record.

Recommendations

A multi-step approach to the neurologic care of reproductive-age women will ensure ethical care, optimal medical management, minimization of risk in future pregnancy, and avoidance of legal liability.

Shared decision-making

The shared decision-making model provides an individualized approach to informed consent. Rather than focusing solely on a discussion of the risks and benefits of treatment, the shared decision-making model takes into consideration a woman's values, beliefs, and priorities. The physician and patient may have differing opinions when it comes to medical decision-making in the context of a potential pregnancy. Conflict may arise when the physician either does not share a woman's values or strongly disagrees with the patient's choices. This conflict may lead to either subtle or overt coercion to select the treatment plan the physician prefers. Only by clarifying the woman's expectations, goals for care, and risk tolerance can a mutually acceptable treatment plan be developed.

Shared decision-making with the patient not only focuses on a treatment decision about the primary neurological condition but also encompasses the totality of the care plan, including the need for family planning, preconception counseling, ongoing monitoring of the patient's condition, and the potential need to alter therapy should pregnancy occur. Physician–patient agreement on all aspects of the care plan maximizes the opportunity for a positive outcome.

Facilitating access to family planning services and preconception counseling

A team-based approach to the care and treatment of women with chronic neurologic disease is ideal to ensure optimal clinical outcomes. The neurologist should recommend that the patient consult with both an obstetrician/gynecologist and a perinatologist to allow for a nuanced discussion of contraceptive choices, timing of pregnancy, and the potential effects of chronic illness and its treatment on future pregnancy. A gynecologist with expertise in family planning can provide counseling about options for contraception, expected efficacy of a chosen method, the importance of compliance, and the need for follow-up to address any concerns or potential changes to the chosen contraceptive method. A perinatologist can discuss the optimal timing of pregnancy with the patient, considering the patient's underlying condition and current treatment plan. In some cases, it may be advisable for the woman to meet with an infertility specialist where either the condition or treatment might impact fertility or there are age-related concerns in the timing of pregnancy.

An important aspect of counseling is a discussion of access to abortion services should that be a possible future consideration. In the current legal landscape, a woman's decision to terminate her pregnancy may no longer be an available course of action. With the overturning of *Roe v Wade*, abortion is no longer a constitutionally protected right; the states through their legislatures may determine if and when pregnancy termination is permissible. The Supreme Court decision in *Dobbs v Jackson Women's Health Organization* means that geographic location determines access to abortion services. As of January 2023, abortion is now banned or significantly limited in 14 states.[19] In these states, clinicians may be reluctant to prescribe potentially teratogenic medications where the option for pregnancy termination is no longer available.[20,21]

Documentation of clinical decision-making and patient counseling
Treating chronic neurologic conditions is often a trial-and-error process whose goal is optimal symptom control for the patient. Physicians must thoroughly document the patient's clinical course and the impact of the condition's evolution on treatment decisions, particularly when teratogenic medications are the treatments of choice. The physician should document the clinical decision-making process, including the informed consent process in the form of shared decision-making. This detailed level of documentation should include the justification for the recommendations made as well as the questions the patient asked and the answers provided.

The need for referrals to other specialties such as gynecology for family planning or perinatology should also be included in the clinical notes, and the patient should be provided with appropriate referrals. In the case of contraceptive counseling, depending on the availability of local resources and access to care, it may be necessary for the treating neurologist to initiate conversations around contraception and prescribe oral contraceptives if appropriate. For women desiring long-acting reversible contraception (LARC) or permanent sterilization, consultation with an obstetrician-gynecologist will be necessary and must be arranged as expediently as possible. Communication with consultants and documentation of those conversations will ensure that the patient's entire care team is sending a cohesive message, thereby, increasing the patient's confidence in medical decision-making and promoting treatment adherence.

Patients should be provided with written resources including treatment recommendations and counseling, referrals for consultation, and scheduled follow-up with their treating health care professional. Regular follow-up will help ensure optimal adherence to the overall treatment plan through assessment of issues with disease-specific treatment, continued satisfaction with and use of contraception, decisions to pursue pregnancy, and possible preconception changes in therapy.

SUMMARY

Potential pregnancy is a consideration when determining optimal management for a woman of reproductive age and includes the effect of pregnancy on the disease and of the disease on the pregnancy, both with and without treatment. The shared decision-making model should be utilized when developing a clinical care plan with a focus on the ethical principles of patient autonomy, beneficence, nonmaleficence, and justice. The shared decision-making model, along with appropriately selected treatment and consultation with other relevant clinical services, meets the criteria for the standard of care even when a given treatment plan carries a risk of harm to a future developing fetus. Legal liability will only occur when the standard of care is breached.

CLINICS CARE POINTS

- Care of reproductive-age women necessitates consideration of potential future fertility when considering treatment decisions.
- Many drugs used in the treatment of neurologic conditions have teratogenic potential.
- Use of teratogenic medications in women of reproductive age should be done to minimize risk to a future pregnancy.
- The shared decision-making model is critical in optimizing benefits to the patient and future pregnancy while minimizing risks.

- Adhering to the standard of care involves not only selecting appropriate disease-specific treatment but also initiating consultations with other specialists and providing adequate neurologic follow-up.
- Documentation of all treatment decisions and patient discussions helps establish that the standard of care was met.

DISCLOSURE

Author has nothing to disclose.

REFERENCES

1. Menstruation in girls and adolescents: using the menstrual cycle as a vital sign. Committee Opinion No. 651. American College of Obstetricians and Gynecologists. Obstet Gynecol 2015;126:e143–6.
2. Management of menopausal symptoms. Practice Bulletin No. 141. American College of Obstetricians and Gynecologists. Obstet Gynecol 2014;123:202–16.
3. Long-acting reversible contraception: implants and intrauterine devices. Practice Bulletin No. 186. American College of Obstetricians and Gynecologists. Obstet Gynecol 2017;130:e251–69.
4. Lockwood CJ, Moore T, Copel J, et al. In: *Creasey & Resnick's Maternal-Fetal Medicine: principles and practice*. 9th edition. Philadelphia: Elsevier; 2023. ISBN 978-0-323-82849-9.
5. Sarayani A, Albogami Y, Thai TN, et al. Prenatal exposure to teratogenic medications in the era of Risk Evaluation and Mitigation Strategies. Am J Obstet Gynecol 2022;227(2):263.e1–38.
6. Vargesson N. Thalidomide-induced teratogenesis: history and mechanisms. Birth Defects Res C Embryo Today 2015;105(2):140–56.
7. Kim JH, Scialli AR. Thalidomide: the tragedy of birth defects and the effective treatment of disease. Toxicol Sci 2011;122(1):1–6.
8. Pernia S, DeMaagd G. The new pregnancy and lactation labeling rule. P T 2016; 41(11):713–5.
9. Food and Drug Adminstration (US). Content and format of labeling for human prescription drug and biological products; requirements for pregnancy and lactation labeling. Final rule. Fed Regist 2014;79(233):72064–103.
10. Nelson LS, Loh M, Perrone J. Assuring safety of inherently unsafe medications: the FDA risk evaluation and mitigation strategies. J Med Toxicol 2014;10(2): 165–72.
11. Federal Food, Drug, and Cosmetic Act ("FDCA"), § 505, 21 U.S.C. § 355 (2020). Available at: https://www.govinfo.gov/content/pkg/USCODE-2010-title21/html/USCODE-2010-title21-chap9-subchapV-partA-sec355.htm#:~:text=No%20person%20shall%20introduce%20or,with%20respect%20to%20such%20drug.
12. Boudes PF. Risk evaluation and mitigation strategies (REMSs): are they improving drug safety? A critical review of remss requiring elements to assure safe use (ETASU). Drugs R 2017;17(2):245–54.
13. Choi JS, Koren G, Nulman I. Pregnancy and isotretinoin therapy. CMAJ (Can Med Assoc J) 2013;185(5):411–3.
14. Food and Drug Aministration (US). FDA Risk Evaluation and Mitigation Strategy (REMS) Public Dashboard. 2023. Available at: https://fis.fda.gov/sense/app/ca

606d81-3f9b-4480-9e47-8a8649da6470/sheet/dfa2f0ce-4940-40ff-8d90-d01c19
ca9c4d/state/analysis. Accessed February 12, 2023.

15. Seizures. Clinical updates in women's health care. American College of Obstetricians and Gynecologists 2021;XX:1.

16. Bosak M, Słowik A, Turaj W. Why do some women with epilepsy use valproic acid despite current guidelines? A single-center cohort study. Epilepsy Behav 2019; 98(Pt A):1–5.

17. Beauchamp TL, Childress JF. Principles of biomedical ethics. 8th ed. New York: Oxford University Press; 2019.

18. Position Statement on the Use of Valproate by Women of Childbearing Potential. American Epilepsy Society. 2021. Available at: https://www.aesnet.org/about/about-aes/position-statements/position-statement-on-the-use-of-valproate-by-women-of-childbearing-potential. Accessed February 12, 2023.

19. Tracking the states where abortion is now banned. The New York Times; 2023. Available at: https://www.nytimes.com/interactive/2022/us/abortion-laws-roe-v-wade.html. Accessed February 14, 2023.

20. LaHue SC, Gano D, Bove R. Reproductive rights in neurology—the supreme court's impact on all of us. JAMA Neurol 2022;79(10):961–2.

21. Rubin R. Threats to evidence-based care with teratogenic medications in states with abortion restrictions. JAMA 2022;328(17):1671–3.

Counseling Patients with Neurologic Disabilities

Sasha Alick-Lindstrom, MD, FAES, FAAN, FACNS[a,b,*]

KEYWORDS

• Disability • Neurologic disorders • Medicolegal • Neuroethics • Beneficence
• Autonomy

BURDEN OF NEUROLOGIC DISEASE

Neurologic disorders constitute the most significant cause of disability and the second highest cause of death globally.[1–3] The World Health Organization ranks neurologic disorders as the leading cause of disability-adjusted life years (DALYs). Neurologic disorders also account for about 9 million deaths per year. The largest contributors of neurologic DALYs in 2016 were stroke (42.2%), migraine (16.3%), dementia (10.4%), meningitis (7.9%), and epilepsy (5%). Parkinson's disease, propelled by an increasingly aging population, is the fastest growing neurologic disorder.[1–3]

Although mortality and morbidity rates clearly vary by condition, a constant across conditions is that most people afflicted tend to be from low- and middle-income class groups. Limited resources to cover adequate supplies, medical care, or caregiver needs only serve to compound poor outcomes. Quality of life metrics should also be examined, as improving them is a driving force for medical interventions and prevention strategies.

BACKGROUND

The urgency to develop viable programs and quality alternatives for those living with neurologic conditions has not emerged from a vacuum. In 1893, when Governor William McKinley declared the Ohio Hospital for Epileptics open for patient admissions, it became the first of several specialized epilepsy colonies in the United States, modeled after several similar ones in Europe, such as Bethel in Bielefeld, Germany.[4] Isolation of patients with neurologic disease contributed to the eugenics movement, and by the early 1900s, several states had passed eugenic sterilization laws for individuals with mental disorders. In its infamous 1927 holding in *Buck vs Bell* 274 US 200 (1927),

---

The author has no commercial or financial conflicts of interest to disclose.
No funding sources to report.
[a] Department of Neurology, Peter O'Donnell Jr Brain Institute, UT Southwestern Medical Center, 5323 Harry Hines Boulevard, Dallas, TX 75390, USA; [b] Department of Radiology, Peter O'Donnell Jr Brain Institute, UT Southwestern Medical Center, 5323 Harry Hines Boulevard, Dallas, TX 75390, USA
* Department of Neurology, Peter O'Donnell Jr Brain Institute, UT Southwestern Medical Center, 5323 Harry Hines Boulevard, Dallas, TX 75390.
E-mail address: Sasha.alicklindstrom@utsouthwestern.edu

the United States Supreme Court determined that forced sterilization of intellectually disabled individuals did not violate the Due Process Clause of the Fourteenth Amendment of US Constitution. Progress on social reform was slow to come, but Franklin Delano Roosevelt's signing into law of the Social Security Act in 1935 was the beginning of a process in which the federal government attempted to provide Americans with a social safety net.[5] The Americans with Disabilities Act of 1990 (ADA), signed into law by President George HW Bush, ushered in a new level of legal protection for individuals with disabilities. The ADA is a federal civil rights law that prohibits discrimination against people with disabilities in everyday activities. The ADA prohibits discrimination based on disability just as other civil rights laws prohibit discrimination based on race, color, sex, national origin, age, and religion. The ADA guarantees that people with disabilities have the same opportunities as everyone else to enjoy employment opportunities, purchase goods and services, and participate in state and local government programs.[6]

CASE PRESENTATION AND DISCUSSION

A 25-year-old woman with uncontrolled epilepsy presents to clinic for consultation. She states that she is eager to have a second child, so she wants to get pregnant soon. She is there with her 3-year-old son, and it is evident she drove to the appointment. Laboratory results reveal low serum medication levels, pointing to poor adherence to antiseizure medications. Her last generalized tonic-clonic seizure was 1 week ago while at work. She states that her family told her she experienced her typical postictal aggression and agitation. She admits she forgot to take her morning dose of antiseizure medication that day but she states that she is usually "pretty good" about taking it. She also reports she was recently fired from her job as an administrative assistant for a business employing approximately 200 people because her employer did not want the liability of having a person with epilepsy working in the office.

How Should This Patient Be Counseled?

Several elements of concern must be addressed during this conversation. The first issue to discuss is medication adherence. The physician should inquire in a nonjudgmental manner about the barriers that this patient is experiencing that prevent her from taking her medications regularly. For example, the patient may not have a full understanding about why strict adherence is so critical. This discussion may need to start with basic information about epilepsy and seizure control to ensure the patient understands what seizures are and why deviating from the treatment plan could lead to breakthrough seizures. Over time, clinical and subclinical seizures may take a toll on her memory, mood, and cognition. Then, the physician should explore concrete factors interfering with adherence, such as financial barriers, cognitive impairment, or mental health challenges. As poorly controlled epilepsy puts the patient at risk of sudden unexpected death in epilepsy (SUDEP), the physician should discuss this risk as well. Frequently, physicians avoid difficult conversations so as not to frighten patients, claiming that by not broaching SUDEP they are acting beneficently; however, by failing to educate patients fully, physicians deprive patients of the ability to make fully informed, autonomous decisions. Approximately one in 1000 people with epilepsy succumb to SUDEP each year and suboptimal adherence to treatment puts the patient at risk of dying from this condition.

Second, the physician should not judge the patient's decision to conceive again, as that is her prerogative, but the patient should be counseled that suboptimal adherence and frequent generalized seizures put both her life and the life of her unborn child at risk. Women with epilepsy can experience safe pregnancies with satisfactory outcomes, but preconception planning, optimal seizure control, and folic acid supplementation are critical elements for creating the conditions for a healthy pregnancy. Ensuring that patients understand the basic elements of their medical condition and associated comorbidities, as well as honoring their motivations and goals, should be at the core of every physician–patient relationship. In women of reproductive age, respecting decisional rights includes discussing the interplay of therapeutic choices on pregnancy outcomes, a topic covered in greater detail in the Susan P. Raine's article, "Legal and Ethical Issues in the Neurology of Reproductive Health," in this volume.

Third, the clinician should address that the patient's driving to the appointment with her son in the car. Driving laws vary by state, and only a handful—California, Oregon, Nevada, Delaware, Pennsylvania, and New Jersey—requires mandatory reporting to the Department of Motor Vehicles. In the remaining states, case law has generally required counseling and documentation of the risks associated with driving and the need to abstain from driving until seizure freedom is achieved for a state-specific statutorily defined period.[7–9] This case is even more problematic because the patient is endangering of her 3-year-old child. Should child protective services (CPS) be contacted or is advising her to stop driving until she acts in compliance with state driving laws enough? The issue of whether to involve CPS is a complex one and is beyond the scope of this article. However, state-specific advice should be sought from individuals with local experience. Furthermore, this patient routinely experiences postictal aggression and agitation. Such behavior may impair a person's judgment to such degree that they inflict harm on others, potentially leading to criminal arrest.[10,11] Under such circumstances, if the welfare of a child is judged to be in danger, CPS is bound to become involved. The best way to prevent such dire consequences for the patient and her family is for her to attain seizure control through medication adherence. If she is not rendered seizure-free through medications alone, she should be referred for a comprehensive evaluation for potential surgical and/or neuromodulation interventions. Again, this frequently entails dedicating time, money, and often travel to specialty centers, which may jeopardize the patient's employment prospects, income stream, and medical insurance coverage.

Fourth, the patient was dismissed from her job after experiencing a seizure. Although improved antiseizure medication adherence may have prevented the seizure that led to her termination, a more critical issue is the legality of that termination. Did this patient's employer violate the ADA when terminating her because of an on-the-job seizure? Individuals with epilepsy face unique challenges because a large proportion do not seem to experience a disability interictally, but during and immediately after the seizure, their disability becomes apparent to employers and coworkers alike. People living with epilepsy frequently hide their condition or else risk losing job security and the much-needed health insurance that often comes along with employment in this country.

The US Equal Opportunity Commission (EEOC), the part of the federal government charged with enforcing the ADA, and other workplace antidiscrimination statues issued a guidance in 2013 entitled "Epilepsy in the Workplace and the ADA."[12,13]:

The EEOC, which was amended by the ADA Amendments Act of 2008 (ADAAA), is a federal law that prohibits discrimination against qualified individuals with disabilities. Individuals with disabilities include those who have impairments that substantially limit a major life activity, have a record (or history) of a substantially limiting impairment, or are regarded as having a disability. Title I of the ADA covers employment by private employers with 15 or more employees as well as state and local government employers. Section 501 of the Rehabilitation Act provides

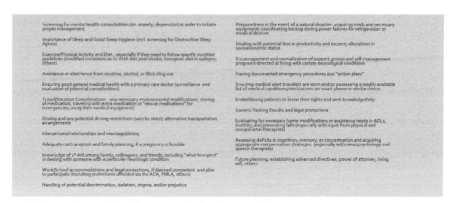

Fig. 1. Lifestyle considerations or modifications to address.

similar protections related to federal employment. In addition, most states have their own laws prohibiting employment discrimination on the basis of disability. Some of these state laws may apply to smaller employers and may provide protections in addition to those available under the ADA.[12]

Although the Supreme Court had initially interpreted the ADA in a way that excluded people with epilepsy from coverage, the ADAAA remedied that issue. The EEOC guidance makes plain that epilepsy qualifies as a disability under the ADAAA:

As a result of changes made by the ADAAA, individuals who have epilepsy should easily be found to have a disability within the meaning of the first part of the ADAs definition of disability because they are substantially limited in neurologic functions and other major life activities (eg, speaking or interacting with others) when seizures occur. In addition, because the determination of whether an impairment is a disability is made without regard to the ameliorative effects of mitigating measures, epilepsy is a disability even if medication or surgery limits the frequency or severity of seizures or eliminates them altogether. An individual with a history of epilepsy (including a misdiagnosis) also has a disability within the meaning of the ADA. Finally, an individual is covered under the third ("regarded as") prong of the definition of disability if an employer takes a prohibited action (eg, refuses to hire or terminates the individual) because of epilepsy or because the employer believes the individual has epilepsy.[12]

The ADAAA prohibits employers from firing individuals because they have epilepsy. Of course, an individual who happens to have epilepsy can be terminated from their job for nonmedical reasons, but neither epilepsy itself nor the need to provide reasonable accommodations to manage the epilepsy can be the reason for terminating an individual. Thus, assuming that the reason for termination was, in fact, epilepsy-related, the patient should be encouraged to file a complaint with the EEOC about her unlawful termination.

Other points to consider when advising patients are listed in **Fig. 1**.

SUMMARY AND FUTURE DIRECTIONS

People living with neurologic conditions may lead full productive lives. Physicians have a duty to educate and counsel their patients, helping them by promoting autonomous decision-making about lifestyle choice and medical care. Neurologists must expand their understanding of how best to manage neurologic disorders to include a thorough consideration of the daily challenges patients with neurologic disease experience as well as taking their patients' intersectional identities, goals, and values into consideration. Clinicians must overcome their own implicit biases when providing care for any individual from historically marginalized groups, including those with disabilities.

CLINICS CARE POINTS

- Neurologic disorders constitute the most significant cause of disability and the second highest cause of death globally.

- People living with neurologic disorders may lead full lives, and accommodations should be pursued, when necessary, so they may remain active participants in their lives and society.

- Health care professionals are obliged physicians to educate and counsel patients, paying with particular attention to patients' desires, beliefs, and perspectives on what constitutes a good quality of life.

- Several considerations to keep in mind and/or address during physician–patient interactions are listed in **Fig. 1**; these topics are broad and many are beyond the scope of this article but may serve as a checklist or guide when dealing with complex cases.

- Neurologist should strive to ensure that care for patients with neurologic disabilities includes a focus on measures that promote patients' integration into society.

REFERENCES

1. Whiteford HA, Ferrari AJ, Degenhardt L, et al. The Global Burden of Mental, Neurological and Substance Use Disorders: An Analysis from the Global Burden of Disease Study 2010. PLoS ONE 2015;10(2):e0116820. https://doi.org/10.1371/journal.pone.0116820.
2. Feigin VL, Vos T, Nichols E, et al. The global burden of neurological disorders: translating evidence into policy. Lancet Neurol 2020;19(3):255–65.
3. Available at: www.who.int/health-topics/brain-health#tab=tab_2.
4. Kissiov D, Dewall T, Hermann B. The Ohio Hospital for Epileptics-the first "epilepsy colony" in America. Epilepsia 2013;54(9):1524–34.
5. Social Security Act (1935) | National Archives. Available at: https://www.archives.gov/milestone-documents/social-security-act.
6. Introduction to the Americans with Disabilities Act | ADA.gov.
7. Kass JS, Rose RV. Driving and Epilepsy: Ethical, Legal, and Health Care Policy Challenges. Continuum (Minneap Minn) 2019;25(2):537–42.
8. Shareef YS, McKinnon JH, Gauthier SM, et al. Counseling for driving restrictions in epilepsy and other causes of temporary impairment of consciousness: how are we doing? Epilepsy Behav 2009;14(3):550–2.
9. Ohtani K, Kawai K. [Driver's License and Welfare Systems for Epilepsy Patients]. Noshinkeigeka 2023;51(1):146–55.
10. McSherry B, Cook M. Seizures, Postictal States and Criminal Responsibility. J Law Med 2022;29(3):707–13.
11. Wortzel HS, Strom LA, Anderson AC, et al. Disrobing associated with epileptic seizures and forensic implications. J Forensic Sci 2012;57(2):550–2.
12. Available at: https://www.eeoc.gov/laws/guidance/epilepsy-workplace-and-ada, Accessed March 20, 2023.
13. Beauchamp T, Childress J. Principles of biomedical ethics. 5th Edition. Oxford University Press; 2001. p. 230–4.

Global Neurology
The Good, the Bad, and the Ugly

James C. Johnston, MD, JD[a,b,*], Thomas P. Sartwelle, BBA, LLB[c],
Mehila Zebenigus, MD[b,d], Berna Arda, MD, MedSpec, PhD[e],
Roy G. Beran, MBBS, MD, MHL[f,g,h] on behalf of the
GlobalNeurology® Publications Committee

KEYWORDS

- Global health programs • Non-government organization
- Low- and middle-income countries • Short-term medical missions
- Global neurology

KEY POINTS

- Neurologists should abandon isolated or short-term medical missions which can and do cause harm, reinforce healthcare disparities, and impede medical care in the regions where it is so desperately needed.
- Integrating neurology with global health requires ethically congruent, multisectoral, interdisciplinary, collaborative partnerships to establish sustainable training programs in low- and middle-income countries.
- Successful training programs align with local needs and conditions, engender support from local health systems, and are amenable to monitoring and evaluation for improved outcomes, efficiency, and growth.
- Healthcare quality must be improved in tandem with quantity while advancing triangular and South-South collaboration to ensure self-sufficiency.

GLOBAL HEALTH: WHY GO BEYOND OUR BORDERS?

The need to be a global consideration is an age old question debated for as long as global health has been a nascent thought during the 16th and 17th centuries age of colonialization. As European countries began to explore new lands like India, China, and the African continent, settlers encountered and returned to Europe with new medical

[a] Auckland, New Zealand and San Antonio, TX, USA; [b] Department of Neurology, Addis Ababa University School of Medicine, Ethiopia; [c] Hicks Davis Wynn, PC, Houston, TX, USA; [d] Yehuleshet Higher Clinic, Addis Ababa, Ethiopia; [e] Department of Medical Ethics, Faculty of Medicine, Ankara University, Turkey; [f] University of New South Wales, Sydney, Australia; [g] Western Sydney University, Sydney, Australia; [h] School of Medicine, Griffith University, Queensland, Australia
* Corresponding author. 17B Farham Street, Auckland 1052, New Zealand; 5290 Medical Drive, San Antonio, Texas 78229, USA
E-mail address: johnston@GlobalNeurology.com

Neurol Clin 41 (2023) 549–568
https://doi.org/10.1016/j.ncl.2023.03.008
0733-8619/23/© 2023 Elsevier Inc. All rights reserved.
neurologic.theclinics.com

maladies motivating physicians to search for cures and their eradication. Since that early period of tropical medicine, the arguments for and against global health have flourished. Those who argue against global health engagement contend that disease and health disparities within one's own borders must be solved before diluting limited resources by exporting health care to other countries. Advocates for global health engagement argue that "local" versus "global" health care is a false dichotomy and focus their attention on the reciprocal benefits of improving health care in both regions. Global health proponents posit engagement as a moral obligation to the international community centered on distributive justice and point to the importance of building capacity to defend against pandemics and minimizing economic risks by improving health on a wider scale, thereby limiting communicable illnesses and ill health.[1–3] Although the argument continues, the reality is that global health programs (GHPs)—government, non-government organizations (NGO), academic, religious, and private for profit—are well entrenched and will not disappear, if for no other reason than the world's intimate interconnectedness and the recently amplified vulnerability to epidemics and pandemics. The real issue in global health is not whether such programs should exist but how to maximize their benefits while mitigating potential harms.

THE RISE OF GLOBAL HEALTH PROGRAMS

Nineteenth-century tropical medicine shifted from missionary physicians and colonial medical services to British and European research institutes and, following widespread government intervention after the United Nation (UN) established World Health Organization (WHO) in 1948, evolved with national and international commissions adopting vertical or parallel programs narrowly targeting specific diseases in one or a few countries (including yaws, tuberculosis, malaria, and poliomyelitis).[4]

Secular missions increased after the 1978 WHO Alma Ata Declaration[5] with the emergence of horizontal primary care models, leading to predominantly NGO or government affiliated programs in the 1980s to 1990s. These have expanded to specialty programs, many embracing elements of both approaches[6,7] and were labeled "global health," a term eluding precise definition[8–14] but promoting the mission to improve health[15] within and among countries[16] by eliminating inequities,[17] addressing social determinants of health,[18] and encompassing endeavors such as security and diplomacy.[19,20]

The two decades preceding the 2019 Severe Acute Respiratory Syndrome Coronavirus 2 (SARS-CoV-2) pandemic witnessed an unprecedented expansion of GHPs, attributable to a constellation of historical, economic, cultural, and religious influences in the milieu of globalization and heightened awareness of health care disparities,[21] accelerated by the United Nations Millennium Declaration 2000[22] and later its 2030 Agenda for Sustainable Development (Agenda).[23] North American academic institutions experienced a more than 10-fold increase in GHPs during the first decade of the millennium,[24,25] leading to some form of global health education in 146 of 153 (95%) surveyed medical schools,[26] with one-third of graduates participating in global health activities.[27]

These GHPs are often fragmented, vertically oriented, lack common standards and competencies, and are predicated on unregulated short-term medical missions (STMMs),[28] an appellation lacking universal definition but viewed as isolated visits from a high-income country (HIC) to a low- or middle-income country (LMIC) for a few days or weeks, exclusive of disaster or conflict services, military practices, or compensated relief missions.[29–32]

STMMs are highly beneficial to the sending institution, providing a heightened profile in academic circles, generating novel research data and, most importantly, securing a share of the widespread global health funding from governments, foundations, and philanthropic organizations.33 These missions are often not aligned with host community needs and preferences,[34–37] operate without standards or accountability,[38,39] generally fail to provide any substantive benefit to the host nation and, in fact, can and do cause actual harm, reinforcing health care disparities by impeding medical care in the very regions it is most needed.[40–44]

Early critics described volunteer doctors turning up *"to do good"* as undermining health care in the community, engaging in inappropriate treatment, with ignorance of local diseases, culture, and language.[45] Others noted that locals were used as *"experimental fodder"* to improve visitor skills.[46] Isolated visits were described as *"nothing more than a glorified form of tourism wrapped in a veneer of altruism, with no sustainable benefits for the receiving communities."*[47]

Although there may be some benefit to select isolated missions in particular settings, notably conflict or disaster relief, or surgical programs engaging in capacity building, a growing body of literature underscores the ethical challenges and legal concerns related to STMMs. However, this literature is limited by the paucity of evidence on prevalence, patient safety, mission impact, and regulation due to the absence of universal guidelines, standards, or accountability.[48,49]

ETHICAL CHALLENGES LEADING TO HARM

The primary goal for any GHP engagement must be improvement of the health and well-being of the host—the individuals and communities that have invited the participants. The visiting health care participants benefit by gaining awareness of global health issues, enjoying travel excursions to exotic locales, advancing clinical skills, enhancing resumes, and the professional and self-satisfaction from tending to those in need. This "experience" is heavily one-sided, and each GHP is also burdened with philosophical, ethical, and legal challenges that must be foremost in the minds of each program participant.[50–52]

These challenges run the gamut, many stemming from the misguided perception that "something is better than nothing," an understandably naive response to the overwhelming poverty in developing regions. They may be merged into a few recurrent themes documented in hundreds of studies, reports, and surveys, including a literature review of 230 articles spanning a 25-year period, numerous anecdotal accounts, and the GlobalNeurology® Partners' experiences, broadly characterized as causing harm to patients and the host community, reinforcing health care disparities, and wasting valuable resources.[53–62]

Accurate diagnoses and appropriate treatment recommendations require knowledge of indigenous diseases, an understanding of the local health system, recognition of language barrier limitations, and a contextual appreciation of social, cultural, economic, and political situations.[63]

Physicians lacking training or experience in resource-limited settings may therefore be ill-suited to provide effective, meaningful care by failing to recognize how well-intentioned recommendations may be inefficient, culturally inappropriate, resource incompatible, and in conflict with the local standard of care. Their care may undermine the host and set the stage for harmful practices.

The physician may view STMMs as an opportunity to perform techniques or procedures beyond what would be permissible at home or may simply feel compelled to act due to overwhelming needs and limited or absent supervision. In one study of 223 respondents, one-half reported being asked to perform beyond the scope of their training, and over 60% of those surveyed admitted doing so.[64] Practicing beyond the scope of one's training is an unethical and harmful practice, unacceptable outside of exigent circumstances such as humanitarian crises. It may lead to malpractice claims or more serious consequences, although such consequences are uncommon in an underprivileged setting with limited regulatory enforcement.[65]

Isolated missions disrupt medical care by requiring usually overburdened local staff to contend with cultural, social, and language barriers while orienting visitors to clinical activities, resource limitations, and personal matters, such as transportation, accommodation, food, and safety issues. Visitors are more often a burden than a help, but hosts may be too polite to object and may continue hosting out of a sense of duty or hope for future support.

Social media may further perpetuate inequities and harm the host through untruthful or misleading reports such as fictitious stories of donations or solicitations for funds based on specious claims of humanitarian work years after a single visit.[51,66] As stated by one global health expert:

Credentialed doctors routinely parachute into poor countries for medical missions that completely disregard local laws and conditions. People think they are doing good, and they have no idea how much harm they can cause. And people back home in the US are often complicit, because when these volunteers write blogs or post videos to share their exploits, 'They're celebrated.'[67]

The literature is replete with examples of poor quality or harmful patient care and the negative impact of STMMs on host communities.[68,69] As summed up by one African hospital staff member, "*I've never seen the contribution, they only waste our time.*"[52] There are nonclinical acts, not always recorded in the literature, revealing the exploitive or "ugly" side of global health. For example, publishing staged photographs of Ethiopian neurologists without permission to solicit donations and failing to account for those funds. Or demanding a host send an invitation letter requesting a grand rounds lecture to surreptitiously provide "justification" for grant-funded vacation travel.

From a practical standpoint, the multiple billions volunteers spend every year traveling the world for a "meaningful" global health experience may be better spent on critical infrastructure and training local health care workers.[70] A 10-person medical team spent USD 30,000 on travel and lodging for one trip to Ghana, half the cost of building a 30-bed hospital.[71] The amount spent on team T-shirts for a visiting delegation would have funded a First Aid station for a year.[72] Misuse of grant money diverts funds that would otherwise aid target countries.[73]

GUIDELINES TO MITIGATE THE HARM

An increasing number of organizations have published guidelines, position statements, and directives to mitigate these STMM harms,[74] and whether based on ethical concerns, guiding ethical principles, a practical view of visitor–host relationships, or more commonly a combination thereof, most share a pervasive disregard for host input that violates traditional bioethical principles and eviscerates the intent, goals, and sustainability of global health engagement.[75–84]

A 2018 review of 27 guidelines,[85] including the Working Group on Ethics and Guidelines for Global Health Training,[86] demonstrated a broad consensus on ethical principles for STMMs, yet the majority (23 of 27) failed to consider host views and almost half never called for or consistently engaged with a host.[87] The American College of Physicians Position Paper,[88] which failed to include a single author from a LMIC, and the Brocher Declaration,[89] authored by an offshoot group from the Consortium of Universities for Global Health,[90] itself criticized for neglecting the South,[91] endorse commendable ethical principles despite promoting STMMs, but they discount reciprocity, downgrade capacity building, and conflate sustainability goals with veritable sustainability. A 2023 review of 35 studies extracted seven core principles aligned with most other ethically driven position statements, but less than half of these studies reported collaboration with the host communities.[92]

A systematic review of 17 studies from the perspective of almost 400 hosts in 25 LMICs corroborated this overriding failure to include the target countries' views, while noting the hosts' preferences for longitudinal relationships based on communication, mutuality, and reciprocity, leading the investigators to emphasize the importance of formalized partnerships with collaboration and predeparture training.[93]

These guidelines and statements are predominantly iterations of bedrock ethical principles that should underscore every physician's behavior such as working to improve health by addressing host-defined needs, demonstrating cultural respect, minimizing burdens, engaging in predeparture preparation, and not practicing beyond the scope of training.[94] However, the impact of these principles on STMMs is questionable.[87] Evidence suggests that most guidelines are not followed in practice,[93] which is not surprising as methods of regulation, reporting, and enforcement do not exist.[87,95,96]

Despite these limitations, there are calls for more guidelines, more mandates, and more position statements. One review suggested, *"Clear guidelines are needed to create global standards to ensure that the services delivered are beneficial not only to patients, but also more broadly to the healthcare systems of recipient countries."*[62] Another concluded, *"There was a need to draft a code of practice creating guidelines that better integrate host country perspectives."*[97]

The concept of a universally acceptable guideline is laudable but may not be possible. Guidelines must be tailored to ensure sociocultural alignment and integration with economic priorities and should address the needs of the local health system, which differ among countries and may vary within different regions of the same country. Guidelines must comport with specific characteristics of the visiting team, whether NGO, university, government, or religious organization, and whether medical or surgical. They need to address the scope of the mission, mutually agreed on goals, the background and training level of participants, and associated collaborative partners.

There are core principles applicable to all organizations, specialties, and regions that may be reduced to a universal directive, departing from STMMs and underscoring the importance of long-term collaboration with capacity building and reciprocity:

There must be an ethically-congruent collaborative approach with proper contextual preparation and training, focusing on the hosts' needs, addressing those needs in written agreements engaging all parties, recognizing and accounting for the disparity in relationships between partners, to establish realistic and mutually agreed upon long term sustainable goals that are designed to advance patient care, physician training, and medical research, focusing on priorities of the South, with transparency and accountability, ensuring full reciprocity, and encouraging triangular and South-South cooperation, with definitive plans for self-sufficiency.[98]

This overarching guide may be refined to meet the needs of individual professional societies and, with effective oversight and regulatory enforcement, would spell the end of many harmful practices. Guidelines should comport with the UN Strategic Development Programme 2022 to 2025.[99] The literature highlights governing options, but further discussion is beyond the scope of this article.[58,100]

LEGAL CONCERNS

This article is limited to reviewing a few legal concerns affecting visitors engaging in missions.[101] GHPs are obligated to abide by host country laws and regulations that are applicable to the program's form of organization.[102] It is incumbent on each program participant or visitor to comply with the host country's legal and regulatory framework. Too often visitors fail to inquire about the situation, disregard the requirements, or presume the laws will not be enforced, expecting the host to assume responsibility and provide blanket protection.

Host country laws that should be considered vary by country but span from entry visa regulations to rules governing patient interactions such as informed consent standards and medical records requirements. Practitioners should be aware of and abide by the relevant laws when visiting a host country and not assume LMICs lack regulatory infrastructure. In fact, it is instructive to review a commonplace example demonstrating that LMICs may have robust medical practice laws.

Patient confidentiality—grounded in ethics, developed in common law, and later codified[103]—is a core principle of medical practice steadfastly protected in developed countries.[104] Visitors presuming confidentiality to be a trivial matter in LMICs are bound to run afoul of the law and place their hosts in legal jeopardy. In Ethiopia, for example, the *Medical Ethics for Doctors* regulations include a "medical secrecy" section stating, in part, "*The doctor shall maintain her/his professional secrecy in respect for all matters . . . in the course of her/his duties to the patients.*"[105] This is enforceable through the Health Professionals Ethics Committee[106] established pursuant to the Food, Medicine, and Health Care Administration and Control Authority (FMHACA) Council of Ministers Regulations,[107] which separately has explicit confidentiality regulations[108] with authority to propose sanctions for unethical or substandard conduct ranging from suspension of licensure to criminal charges.[109]

Medical licensure

Many countries require volunteer physicians to possess temporary or provisional licensure, registration, or approval from the local Ministry of Health or professional licensing board. Ethiopia,[110,111] Kenya,[112] and Tanzania[113] have licensure requirements for foreign volunteers; Uganda[114] and Rwanda[115] require a provisional license; Zimbabwe[116] requires a letter of permission; Nigeria[117] invokes criminal punishment for foreigners practicing without registration; the Caribbean Association of Medical Councils has varying requirements[118]; and the Association of Southeast Asian Nations requires licensure.[119] Visitors ignoring local licensing regulations place the host at risk of sanctions and may themselves be subject to the vagaries of a foreign court system with the potential for criminal or civil complaints.[120] Following applicable licensing laws represent the hallmark of an ethical, responsible engagement, repeatedly supported in guidelines and position papers.[121]

Medical Malpractice

Medical malpractice is an increasing concern worldwide due to an expanding litigation culture leading to an increasing number of claims against physicians.[122] There are limited case reports because the hurdles of accessing courts in many jurisdictions lead to informal settlement. Even in a resource limited nation such as Ethiopia, with a complicated civil law system allowing claims in tort, contract, or criminal law, there are lawyers advertising to accept cases. Malpractice claims in Ethiopia have increased over the past decade.[123–125] This legal landscape is particularly concerning when visitors with inadequate local knowledge and preparation engage in patient care, and host physicians lack experience with the visitors' procedures or treatment, opening the door for negligence claims against either or both parties. The host faces the greatest risk of sanctions or fines. In Ethiopia, the FMHACA specifically states that an institution accommodating a visiting professional must "*bear civil responsibility for any damages caused by health services provided by the professional.*"[126] Some jurisdictions have a liability exemption for volunteer acts carried out in good faith, if the provider is *"properly licensed and certified to perform the task required,"* and there was no recklessness, criminal act, or use of drugs or alcohol, but this protection may be limited to citizens, not foreign nationals.[127]

Donations

Donations of medical equipment and pharmaceutical supplies are also problematic.[120] There are special concerns with equipment—whether it is contextually appropriate, relevant to local needs, able to be properly maintained, and if accepting the equipment places the host at risk of violating importation, taxation, and registration laws. Pharmaceutical donations raise complex regulatory issues intersecting multiple legal frameworks in the United States and host countries that are best managed through legal guidance in both countries. There are ethical and medical concerns with visitors importing the latest antiseizure medications or a supply of botulinum toxin and left in the hands of local medical staff unfamiliar with their proper use and potential complications, including interactions with traditional treatments. Local staff is also left to manage a difficult situation when the limited supplies run out.

Many concerns would be preempted by directing inquiries to the host in advance to ensure an agreed on donation complies with all local laws and regulations. The WHO recognized that donations can *"constitute an added burden to the recipient health care system"* and in coordination with several international health organizations, the UN, and the World Bank, established specific guidelines addressing the problem,[128] which comport with earlier policies that donors must *"respect the laws, regulations, and administrative procedures of the recipient country."*[129]

Medical Research

Medical research endeavors, driven by economic or academic interests that risk exploiting vulnerable populations, raise myriad complex ethical and legal concerns, spanning informed consent through to data extraction and authorship agreements. Extensive international policies, statements, and guidelines address many of these research concerns and are designed to ensure an ethical balance of interests.[130,131] Researchers from abroad and their local hosts should consult relevant standards in both the sending and host countries before embarking on research ventures.[132]

WHAT ABOUT GLOBAL NEUROLOGY?

The emergence of global neurology, at a time of heightened interest in global health and with neurological diseases acknowledged to be a pressing concern in LMICs, provides a unique opportunity for neurologists to adopt best practices. These should emanate from global health colleagues, leverage the pandemic disruptions, and focus on improved access to sustainable neurological care for the world's most vulnerable patients.

An Emerging Field

US neurologists have embraced global health. Some residency training programs offer clinical electives in LMICs. Numerous funding opportunities for global health research and a wide range of part and full-time career options have emerged.[133] The American Academy of Neurology (AAN) established a Global Health Section, sponsors a monthly Global Health webinar, highlights Global Neurology Research Updates, coordinates

Global Neurology lectures at annual meetings, and publishes a 'Global Neurology' section in the flagship journal.[134] It is one of six affiliated regional neurological associations holding membership in the World Federation of Neurology under the auspices of "Global Neurology."[135] By endorsing global neurology, the AAN is well positioned to coordinate meaningful guidelines and position statements to advance care where it is most needed.

Integrating Neurology with Global Health

The fundamental goal of global health is to reduce or eliminate health inequities.[136] Inequities are varied and attributable to diverse factors specific to particular regions and are shaped by local values and ideologies. The underlying commonality is a lack of access to health-related services, fostering ill-health and exacerbating poverty in a mutually reinforcing cycle with multiple interconnected, contributory, and reciprocal factors, including the negative impact of poverty on health, resulting in excessive maternal, neonatal, and childhood morbidity and mortality, ongoing high rates of infectious diseases, and the greatest burden today, which is "[untreated] *non-communicable diseases that are forcing millions of people into poverty annually.*"[137]

The most disconcerting noncommunicable diseases are the neurological conditions, such as stroke, epilepsy, and dementia, which have an extraordinarily high rate of morbidity, afflicting millions of people, resulting in both poor cognition and physical impairment. Such diseases render the affected individuals unable to reach their full potential, with lost income and fewer opportunities, leading to increased vulnerability, marginalization, and exclusion, resulting in overwhelming psychological suffering as well as medical and social needs.[65,138] These neurological disorders, disproportionately increasing in incidence in LMICs,[139,140] profoundly impact the economic, social, and political stability of the country and represent the *"greatest threat to global public health."*[141]

This is precisely why the Agenda[142] Sustainable Development Goal 3 (*"ensure healthy lives and promote well-being at all ages"*), subsuming nine substantive and four secondary targets, underpinned by the goal of advancing *inter alia* "*access to quality essential healthcare services,*"[143] aims to "*reduce by one-third premature mortality from non-communicable diseases.*"[144] This goal aligns with the WHOs recently enacted Intersectoral Global Action Plan on Epilepsy and Other Neurological Disorders 2022 to 2031 (IGAP).[145]

The remaining questions are where to start and how to most effectively advance access to neurological services.

Where to Start?

The Agenda provides guidance on where to start: *"reach the furthest behind first,"*[146] meaning the least developed nations,[147] which are predominantly in sub-Saharan Africa (SSA), on a continent of 1.5 billion people harboring one-quarter of the global burden of disease, less than 2% of the world's health care professionals, and consuming less than 1% of the global health care expenditure.[148] These regions have inherently vulnerable populations and present special challenges requiring particular attention[149] to ensure that each person receives "*the highest attainable standard of health as a fundamental right.*"[150]

How to Improve Access to Neurological Care?

Neurologists should abandon STMMs, which are a waste of limited health care resources expended on ephemeral efforts providing no enduring solution. GlobalNeurology recommended this sweeping change over a decade ago, drawing vehement opposition from some US academic neurologists[151–155]; however, our position was later supported by global neurology experts adopting a long term collaborative approach in developing successful neurology programs in Haiti[156] and Zambia.[157]

The single most effective method for improving access to sustainable neurological care is to increase the recruitment, development, training, and retention of neurologists and related health care workers in LMICs.[158] This approach provides a cross-cutting impact on the myriad substantial impediments inherent in resource-limited regions,[138] aligns with the Agenda,[159] is supported by the WHO,[160] and is endorsed through the IGAP objectives and global targets.[161]

The global neurologist must enter a long-term, ethically congruent, collaborative partnership with an established health system or medical school wishing to initiate or advance neurological services. Such a partnership can lay the foundations for a training program comporting with local needs and conditions that is supported by the local health system, and is amenable to monitoring and evaluation for improved outcomes, efficiency, and growth.

There must be a willingness to participate in a network of multisectoral, interdisciplinary partnerships, established deliberately, ethically, and collaboratively, focusing on capacity building to achieve self-sufficiency. Such programs must train local physicians working in local conditions to treat local diseases. This approach improves care, services, and education while protecting fragile, overwhelmed medical systems and vulnerable populations. It avoids donor-based protection policies that provide no substantive benefit and are destined to fail.[162]

Multisectoral Triangular Collaboration

The academic programs focusing on unidirectional propagation or bilateral engagements with limited reciprocity may not be interested in a multi-institutional, multisectoral plan with triangular or multilateral collaboration facilitating South-South initiatives, yet such a plan is essential to advance the cross-cutting nature of the Agenda, bringing modern sustainable health care to the areas of greatest need—the "furthest behind."[163]

Multi-institutional involvement is fundamental to successful development of a training program. Different institutions offer complementary services, strengthening the host program, leading to specialized clinics and expanded research opportunities. However, this approach requires careful attention to potential hurdles such as redundant services, failed reciprocity, or one university adopting a proprietary stance.

GlobalNeurology® illustrates the importance of adopting a highly collaborative and multi-institutional approach. This NGO is accredited by the WHO, in Special Consultative Status with the UN Economic and Social Council, and represents an international partnership[164] of neurologists, neurosurgeons, and neuroethicists, with a mission to advance sustainable neurological care in resource limited settings. It holds a long-standing relationship with the Addis Ababa University (AAU) Department of Neurology Residency Training Program ("Program") in Ethiopia, which provides a backdrop for some of the views, opinions, and examples in this article.

In 2006, Ethiopian neurologist Professor Guta Zenebe spearheaded the Program, backed by AAU and the Ethiopian Ministry of Health, with strong international support from both the Mayo Clinic led by Dr James Bower and GlobalNeurology® led by Dr James C. Johnston, and later collaborations with several universities, NGOs, and private institutions. The AAU Department of Neurology governs the Program, which is now self-sufficient, having graduated 81 board-certified adult neurologists,[165] most practicing in Ethiopia and, more importantly in a nation of 120 million people where there may never be enough neurologists, teaching the primary care physicians how to manage common neurological conditions. The Program also trains physicians from other African nations, thereby taking an innovative lead in triangular and South–South cooperation.[23]

The following examples highlight a few GlobalNeurology® engagements with the Program during a brief window before the pandemic, noting that all activities were requested by, coordinated with, and approved through the AAU Department of Neurology. These very fundamental considerations underscore the importance of communication and addressing the hosts' needs.

The Partners provided regularly scheduled on-site teaching, remaining available remotely between trips, and coordinating neurologists from the European Union, Israel, Norway, the United Kingdom, and the United States to teach. Global-Neurology® developed collaborations with multiple universities to advance the Program including University of Siena, Italy; University of Bergen, Norway; University of Cape Town, South Africa; University of Geneva, Switzerland; and Ankara University, Turkey. These were established for specific reasons. For example, the University of Siena provided an annual neurophysiology fellowship. Clinical rotations were provided in Australia, South Africa, and Turkey. An Israeli neurology team was invited to establish a pediatric epilepsy clinic in northern Ethiopia. Other capacity building efforts included mentoring research projects and supporting other universities, institutions, or NGOs, developing an electroencephalogram (EEG) technician school in northern Ethiopia, a pediatric nursing forum, and a rehabilitation program.

GlobalNeurology® represents the Program at various WHO, UN, and other international meetings. Advocacy is important, and presenting the Program at annual global conferences builds relationships, which may lead to partnerships, resident scholarships, or equipment donations.

This comprehensive, collaborative approach is not only successful, as evidenced by the Ethiopian Program, but critical for advancing neurology in SSA, where the current ratio of one neurologist for every 3 to 5,000,000 people is far below the WHO recommended ratio of 1:100,000 and the HIC ratio of 4.75:100,000 people.[166]

South–South Collaboration

South–South cooperation is vital to improving health care access in a sustainable cross-cutting manner leading to self-sufficiency.[167] A quintessential example is the highly successful and innovative African Paediatric Fellowship Programme directed by Professor Jo Wilmshurst at the University of Cape Town, South Africa.[168] This program includes training collaborations with 15 African countries. Referring partner centers recruit trainees for targeted training in critical areas of pediatric health care. Training is predominantly undertaken in South Africa, but end-stage capacity building is finally being reached and other training hubs are being established across the continent, most recently in Kenya. There is a 95% retention rate of trainees returning to deliver care and take on leadership roles in their home setting.[169] This program is crucial to the development and expansion of child neurology and other pediatric specialties throughout Africa.

Quality in Tandem with Quantity

The quality of health care is fundamental to health equity and must be improved in tandem with quantity as poor quality obviates the benefits of increased access, wastes valuable resources, and causes actual harm through inverse, unsafe, fragmented, and misdirected care.[162] Poor quality care is now a greater contributor to mortality than limited access to health care. The Global Health Commission on High-Quality Health Systems concluded that 5.7 million people in LMICs die every year from poor quality health care compared with 2.9 million dying from lack of access.[170–172] Improving quality requires input from multiple, diverse stakeholders in each country and necessitates reforms impacting all levels of public and private health services. There is a need to address governance structures, service delivery, educational processes, and accountability methods, representing an extraordinarily complex topic that is beyond the scope of this article.[173]

Good Intentions Not a Substitute for Ethical Actions

The academic global neurology rotations which send trainees to an LMIC for a few days or weeks annually are tantamount to repetitive isolated missions and fail to provide any substantial capacity-building. This approach represents a paternalistic view of global health development.

In a recent survey of neurology residents who completed a *"global health experience,"* the majority reported gaining improved clinical and examination skills, gaining an understanding of different health systems, and "more judicious use of resources upon returning to the United States," leading to the conclusion, *"Global health electives had a positive impact on neurology trainees."*[174] However, did anyone survey the hosts? What did they receive?

Arguments that 83% of the trainees reported a *"deeper commitment to underserved populations"*[65] may suggest good intentions, but that neither substitutes for ethical actions nor benefits the host. A recent AAN Global Health blog underscored this survey with suggestions to *"create a platform by which students, trainees, and faculty interested in having an education experience in another country may be able to find a list of rotations or observerships."*[175] Again, the intentions are undoubtedly noble, but this approach is antithetical to ethical global health endeavors.

The focus must be on the needs of the host which should be defined by the host. Rotations or observerships may have a role in established host programs, but this will only be the case if there exists a collaborative institutional engagement with mutual benefit and reciprocity.[176,177]

SUMMARY

Several million words concerning global health have been written in books, journal articles, professional society recommendations, consortium position papers, and by government and NGOs involved in global health endeavors. Virtually every conceivable scenario has been analyzed. The literature is far too dense to cover within the confines of this introductory article, aside from providing a few references and identifying readily available resources to promote reconsideration of what is available.[178] Global health services can be enhanced to accommodate the real needs of the recipients of the largess that achieves more than the personal gratification of the providers.

In reality, global health ethics—the framework for advancing health equity—despite the millions of words already written on this topic, the newly invented terminology, the intricate moral value arguments, the deepened ethical understandings, and the multiplicity of guidelines, can be summarized easily through words written more than 250 years ago by the German Enlightenment philosopher Immanuel Kant: *"So act that your principle of action might safely be made a law for the whole world."*

The English puritan preacher John Bunyan, famous as the author of the allegory *The Pilgrim's Progress*, unintentionally summarized the totality of global health ventures, from the past to well into our future, when he wrote: *"You have not lived today until you have done something for someone who can never repay you."* This should be the guiding ethical principle for each individual participating in any global health endeavor.

AUTHOR CONTRIBUTIONS

The authors contributed equally to the research, development, writing, review, and approval of the content.

DECLARATION OF CONFLICTING INTERESTS

The authors have no competing interests to declare.

FUNDING

The authors received no financial support for this article.

ACKNOWLEDGMENTS

The authors gratefully acknowledge the scholarly and editorial contributions of the following individuals: (i) Professor Guta Zenebe, Department of Neurology, Addis Ababa University School of Medicine, Ethiopia and Founder, Yehuleshet Specialty Clinic and Yehuleshet Hospital, Addis Ababa, Ethiopia. (ii) Professor Jo Wilmshurst, Head of Paediatric Neurology, Red Cross Memorial Children's Hospital, Neuroscience Institute, University of Cape Town, South Africa; and Director of the African Paediatric Fellowship Program, University of Cape Town, South Africa.

REFERENCES

1. Ruchman SG, Singh P, Stapleton A. Why US health care should think globally. AMA J Ethics 2016;18(7):736–42.
2. Ekmekci PE, Arda B. Luck egalitarianism, individual responsibility and health. Balkan Med J 2015;32:244–54.
3. World Health Organization. Global health ethics: key issues. Geneva, Switzerland: World Health Organization; 2015.
4. Greenwood A, editor. Beyond the state: the colonial medical service in British Africa. University of Manchester, UK: Manchester University Press; 2019.
5. World Health Organization. Declaration of Alma Ata 1978. International conference on primary health care, Alma Ata. Geneva: World Health Organization; 1978.
6. Mills A. Mass campaigns versus general health services: what have we learnt in 40 years about vertical versus horizontal approaches? Bull WHO 2005;83(4): 315–6.
7. Msuya J. Horizontal and vertical delivery of health services: what are the trade-offs? The World Bank 1818H Street NW, Washington, DC 20433.
8. Koplan JP, Bond TC, Merson MH, et al. Towards a common definition of global health. Lancet 2009;373(9679):1993–5.
9. Institute of Medicine (US). Committee on the US commitment to Global Health. The US commitment to global health: recommendations for the public and private sectors. Washington DC: National Academies Press (US); 2009.
10. Taylor S. Global health: meaning what? BMJ Glob Health 2018;3:e000842.
11. Sheikh K, Schneider H, Agyepong IA, et al. Boundary-spanning: reflections on the practices and principles of global health. BMJ 2016;1:e00058.
12. Fried LP, Bentley ME, Buekens P, et al. Global health is public health. Lancet 2010;375:535–7.
13. Kuhlmann AS, Iannotti L. Resurrecting international and public in global health: has the pendulum swung too far? Am J Publ Health 2014;104(4):583–5.

14. King NB, Koski A. Defining global health as public health somewhere else. BMJ Glob Health 2020;5:e002172.
15. World Health Organization. Constitution, preamble, at 1. Geneva: World Health Organization; 1948. Improving health does not simply refer to the absence of disease but a "state of complete physical, mental, and social well-being.
16. Amouzou A, Kozuki N, Gwatkin DR. Where is the gap? The contribution of disparities within developing countries to global inequities in under-five mortality. BMC Publ Health 2014;14:216.
17. McCartney G, Popham F, McMaster R, et al. Defining health and health inequalities. Publ Health 2019;172:22–30.
18. Frank J, Abel T, Campostrini S, et al. The social determinants of health: time to re-think? Int J Environ Res Public Health 2020;17(16):5856.
19. Kevany S. James Bond and global health diplomacy. Int J Health Policy Manag 2015;4(12):831–4.
20. Michaud J, Kates J. Global health diplomacy: advancing foreign policy and global health interests. Glob Health Sci Pract 2013;1(1):24–8.
21. Merson MH, Page KC. The dramatic expansion of university engagement in global health: implications for US policy. A Report of the CSIS Global Health Policy Center, 2009 at 2.
22. United Nations. United nations millennium declaration. New York: United Nations; 2000.
23. United Nations. Transforming our world: the 2030 agenda for sustainable development A/RES/70/1. Geneva: United Nations; 2015.
24. Merson MH. University engagement in global health. N Engl J Med 2014;370:1676–8.
25. Khan OA, Guerrant R, Sanders J, et al. Global health education in US medical schools. BMC Med Educ 2013;13(1).
26. Available at: https://www.aamc.org/data-reports/curriculum-reports/interactive-data/curriculum-topics-required-and-elective-courses-medical-school-programs. (Accessed January 4, 2023.
27. Medical school graduation questionnaire: 2018 all schools summary report. Association of American Medical Colleges. Available at: https://www.aamc.org/system/files/reports/1/2018gqallschoolssummaryreport.pdf. (Accessed January 4, 2023).
28. Also labeled short-term experiences in global health or STEGH, internships, brigades, global health electives, international rotations, and similar monikers.
29. Arther MAM. Teaching the basics: core competencies in global health. Inf Dis Clin NA 2011;25(2):347–58.
30. Brewer TF. From boutique to basic: a call for standardized medical education in global health. Med Ed 2009;43(10):930–3.
31. Battat R. Global health competencies and approaches in medical education. BMC Med 2010;10:94.
32. Kerry VB, Ndung'u T, Walensky RP, et al. Managing the demand for global health education. PLoS Med 2011;8(11):e1001118.
33. Supra note 24. See also Crump JA, Sugarman J. Ethics and best practice guidelines for training experiences in global health. Am J Trop Med Hyg 2010;83(6):1178–82.
34. Rozier MD, Lasker JN, Compton B. Short-term volunteer health trips: aligning host community preferences and organizer practices. Glob Health Action 2017;10(1):1267957.

35. Lu PM, Mansour R, Qui MK, et al. Low and middle income country host perceptions of short-term experiences in global health: a systematic review. Acad Med 2021;96(3):460–9.

36. Lasker JN. Global health volunteering: understanding organizational goals. Voluntas Int J Voluntary Nonprofit Organ 2016;27:574–94.

37. Lasker JN. Hoping to help: the promises and pitfalls of global health volunteering (the culture and politics of health care work). Ithaca, NY: Cornell University Press; 2016.

38. Maki J, Qualls M, White B, et al. Health impact assessment and short term medical missions: a methods study to evaluate quality of care. BMC Health Serv Res 2008;8:121.

39. Supra notes 36, 37.

40. Johnston J.C., Zebenigus M., on behalf of GlobalNeurology®. United Nations High Level Segment. Geneva, Switzerland. 2016. E/2016/NGO/53.

41. Macfarlane SB, Jacobs M, Kaaya EE. In the name of global health: trends in academic institutions. J Pub Health Policy 2008;29(4):383–401.

42. Martiniuk ALC, Manouchehrian M, Negin JA, et al. Brain gains: a literature review of medical missions to low and middle income countries. BMC Health Serv Res 2012;12:134.

43. Supra note 34. See also Crump J.A. and Sugarman J., Examining the scale and outcomes of global health fellowships in the United States, *JGME*, 4 (2), 2012, 261–262.

44. Melby MK, Loh LC, Evert J, et al. Beyond medical missions to impact-driven short-term experiences in global health (STEGHs): ethical principles to optimize community benefit and learner experience. Acad Med 2016;91(5):633–8.

45. Bishop R, Litch J. Medical tourism can do harm. BMJ 2000;320(7240):1017.

46. Dupuis C. Humanitarian missions in the Third World: a polite dissent. Plast Reconstr Surg 2004;113:433–5.

47. Snyder J, Dharamsi S, Crooks VA. Fly-by medical care: conceptualizing the global and local social responsibilities of medical tourists and physician voluntourists. Glob Health 2011;6(7):1–14.

48. Sykes KJ. Short term medical service trips: a systematic review of the evidence. Am J Publ Health 2014;104(7):e38–48.

49. Supra note 37. See also, Cheng MY, Rodriguez E. Short-term medical relief trips to help vulnerable populations in Latin America. Bringing clarity to the scene. Int J Env Res Pub Health 2019;16:745.

50. Stapleton G, Schroder-Back P, Laaser U, et al. Global health ethics: an introduction to prominent theories and relevant topics. Glob Health Action 2014;7(1):1–7.

51. Supra note 34.

52. Supra note 37.

53. Penney D. Ethical considerations for short-term global health projects. J Midwifery Wom Health 2020;65(6):767–76.

54. Supra note 45.

55. Bezruchka S. Medical tourism as medical harm to the third world: Why? For Whom? Wild Environ Med 2000;11:77–8.

56. Supra note 46.

57. Welling D, Ryan J, Burris D, et al. Seven sins of humanitarian medicine. World J Surg 2010;34:466–70.

58. Supra note 42.

59. Lasker JN, Aldrink M, Balasubramaniam R, et al. Guidelines for responsible short-term global health activities: developing common principles. Glob Health 2018;14(18):1–9.
60. Bauer I. More harm than good? The questionable ethics of medical volunteering and international student placements. Tropical Diseases, Travel Medicine and Vaccines 2017;3(5):1–12.
61. Provenzano AM, Graber LK, Elansary M, et al. Short term global health research projects by US medical students: ethical challenges for partnerships. Am J Trop Med Hyg 2010;83(2):211–4.
62. Roche SD, Ketheeswaran P, Wirtz VJ. International short term medical missions: a systematic review of recommended practices. Int J Public Health 2017;62(1):31–42.
63. Wall A. The context of ethical problems in medical volunteer work. HEC Forum 2011;23:63–79.
64. Doobay-Persaud A, Evert J, DeCamp M, et al. Extent, nature and consequences of performing outside scope of training in global health. Glob Health 2019;15(60):1–11.
65. Id.
66. Tabb Z, Hyle L, Haq H. Pursuit to post: ethical issues of social media use by international medical volunteers. Dev World Bioeth 2021;21(3):102–10.
67. Gostin L. Global Health Law. Harvard University Press; 2014. 9780674728844.
68. Supra notes 53-62.
69. Evert J, Todd T, Zitek P. Do you GASP? How pre-health students delivering babies in Africa is quickly becoming consequentially unacceptable. The Advisor (December 2015) at 61-65.
70. Caldron PH, Impens A, Pavlova M, et al. Economic assessment of US physician participation in short term medical missions. Glob Health 2016;12(45):1–10.
71. Abdullah F. Perspective of West Africa: why bother to 'mission? Arch Surg 2008;143(8):728–9.
72. Montgomery L. Reinventing short-term medical missions to Latin America. J Lat Am Theol 2007;2(2):84–103.
73. On file with authors.
74. Supra note 62, documenting some improvement over the 25 year study period attributable to the Paris Treaty and Accra Accord.
75. Stone GS, Olsen KR. The ethics of medical volunteerism. Med Clin North Am 2016;100:237–46.
76. DeCamp M. Ethical review of global short term medical volunteerism. HEC Forum 2011;23:91–103.
77. Conard CJ, Kahn MJ, DeSalvo KB, et al. Student clinical experiences in Africa: who are we helping? Virtual Mentor 2006;8(12):855–8.
78. Crump JA, Sugarman J. Ethical considerations for short-term experiences by trainees in global health. JAMA 2008;300(12):1456–8.
79. Chiverton A. Ethics of international medical electives in the developing world: helping those in need or helping ourselves? Bioethics 2009;46.
80. Supra note 44.
81. Supra note 62.
82. Lough BJ, Tiessen R, Lasker JN. Effective practices of international volunteering for health: perspectives from partner organizations. Glob Health 2018;14(1):1–11.
83. Loh LC, Cherniak W, Dreifuss BA, et al. Short term global health experiences and local partnership models: a framework. Glob Health 2015;11(1):50.

84. Supra notes 33, 34, 36, 37. See also Infra notes 90, 96.

85. Supra note 59.

86. Supra note 33.

87. Supra notes 37, 59.

88. DeCamp M, Lehmann LS, Jaeel P, et al. Ethical obligations regarding short term global health clinical experiences: an American College of Physicians Position Paper. Ann Int Med 2018;168:651–7.

89. Available at: https://static1.squarespace.com/static/5f2c809ea363711e6b06579c/t/5fbed8403485235c86ad4b93/1606342720768/Brocher+Declaration+Final+ver.pdf. (Accessed January 6, 2023).

90. Prasad S, Aldrink M, Compton B, et al. Global health partnerships and the Brocher Declaration: principles for ethical short-term engagements in global health. Ann Global Health 2022;88(1):1–9, 31.

91. Crane J. Scrambling for Africa? Universities and global health. Lancet 2011; 377(1113):1388–9.

92. Leversedge C, McCullough M, Appiani LMC, et al. Capacity building during short-term surgical outreach trips: a review of what guidelines exist. World J Surg 2023;47(1):50–60.

93. Supra note 35.

94. Taylor RM. Ethical principles and concepts in medicine. Handb Clin Neurol 2013;118:1–9.

95. Rowthorn V, Loh L, Evert J, et al. Not above the law: a legal and ethical analysis of short-term experiences in global health. Ann Glob Health 2019;85(1): 1–12, 79.

96. Caldron PH, Impens A, Pavlova M, et al. A systematic review of social, economic and diplomatic aspects of short term medical missions. BMC Health Serv Res 2015;15:380.

97. Tracey P, Rajaratnam E, Varughese J, et al. Guidelines for short term medical missions: perspectives from host countries. Glob Health 2022;18:19.

98. Johnston J.C., Zebenigus M., on behalf of GlobalNeurology®. Developing and improving healthcare services in resource limited areas. Fifty fifth session of the United Nations Commission for Social Development. New York, NY. 1-10 Feb 2017. E/CN.5/2017/NGO/19.

99. Available at: https://www.undp.org/publications/undp-strategic-plan-2022-2025. (Accessed January 18, 2023).

100. Supra note 95.

101. See generally Gostin LO, Sridhar D. Global health and the law. N Engl J Med 2014;370:1732–40.

102. For example, Ethiopia recently enacted the Organization of Civil Societies Proclamation No. 1113/2019 which covers the duties, taxes, reports, and other government matters impacting NGOs. Available at: https://cof.org/sites/default/files/documents/files/Country-Notes/Nonprofit-Law-in-Ethiopia.pdf.   (Accessed December 19, 2022).

103. Beran R., ed. Legal and forensic medicine. Berlin, Germany: Springer-Verlag Publishing, 2013. Sections V (informed consent) and XV (privacy).

104. Taylor MJ, Wilson J. Reasonable expectations of privacy and disclosure of health data. Med Law Rev 2019;27(3):432–60. See, Hunter v. Mann (1974) 1QB 767.

105. Ethiopian Medical Association. Medical Ethics for Doctors in Ethiopia, Section III, Article 21 .Available at: (https://www.ethiopianmedicalass.org/download/medical-ethics-for-doctors-in-ethiopia-2/). (Accessed January 4, 2023).

106. The mandates of this Committee are set forth by the Food, Medicine, and Healthcare Administration and Control Proclamation No. 661/2009; Food, Medicine, and Healthcare Administration and Control Regulations No. 299/2013 and 189/2009; The FDRE Criminal Code, and the 1960 Civil Code of Ethiopia.

107. Council of Ministers Regulation No. 299/2013. Federal Negarit Gazette, 20th Year No. 11, Addis Ababa, 24 January 2014. Available at: http://www.efda. gov.et/publication/food-medicine-and-healthcare-administration-and-control-councils-of-ministers-regulation-no-299-2013/. (Accessed January 7, 2023).

108. Id. at Chap 2, Articles 744, 771.

109. Supra note 107 at Chap 2, Article724.

110. Available at: https://www.moh.gov.et/site/Voluntary_Service_Requirement. (Accessed January 15, 2023).

111. Supra note 107, Article 68(3) . . . grants authority to issue a temporary license "when the professional intends to provide health services in short term charitable activities." Also noting section (4) of the same Article holds that the institution which brought the professional "bears civil responsibility for any damages caused by the health service provided by the (visiting) professional."

112. Available at: https://kmpdc.go.ke/foreign-trained-doctors/ with link for temporary licensure. (Accessed January 15, 2023).

113. Available at: https://mct.go.tz/index.php/limited-registrations-foreigners. (Accessed January 15, 2023).

114. Available at: https://umdpc.com/forms.php. (Accessed January 15, 2023).

115. Available at: https://www.rmdc.rw/spip.php?article397. (Accessed January 15, 2023).

116. Available at: https://www.mdpcz.co.zw/the-profession/policies-and-guidelines/. (Accessed January 15, 2023).

117. Available at: https://www.mdcnigeria.org/downloads/guidelines-on-registration. pdf at 20. (Accessed January 15, 2023).

118. Available at: https://www.camcouncils.org/. (Accessed December 15, 2022).

119. Available at: https://asean.org/asean-mutual-recognition-arrangement-on-medical-practitioners/. (Accessed January 15, 2023).

120. Supra note 95.

121. See, e.g., WEIGHT ("comply with licensing standards"), American College of Physicians ("licensing requirements must be adhered to"), Brocher ("A major concern is ignorance or subversion of relevant laws that do exist for instance medical licensure regulations in host countries"), GlobalNeurology® ("comply with licensing regulations in the host country").

122. World Medical Association General Assembly. WMA Statement on Medical Liability. Adopted 2005, reaffirmed 2015, amended 2021. Available at: https://www. wma.net/policies-post/wma-statement-on-medical-liability-reform/. (Accessed January 15, 2023).

123. Wamisho BL, Lidiya MAT, Teklemariam E. Surgical and medical error claims in Ethiopia: trends observed from 125 decisions made by the Federal Ethics Committee for Health Professionals Ethics Review. Medicolegal Bioeth 2019;9:23–31.

124. Melberg A, Teklemariam L, Moland KM, et al. Juridification of maternal deaths in Ethiopia: a study of the Maternal and Perinatal Death Surveillance and Response (MPDSR) system. Health Pol Plann 2020;35(8):900–5.

125. Wamisho BL, Abeje M, Feleke Y, et al. Analysis of medical malpractice claims and measures proposed by the Health Professionals Ethics Federal Committee of Ethiopia: review of three years proceedings. Ethiop Med J 2015;53(Supp 1):1–6.

126. Supra note 107 at Article 68(4).
127. Elgafi S. Medical liability in humanitarian missions. J Humanitarian Assistance 2014.
128. World Health Organization. Guidelines for Medicine Donations. 2010, WHO (ISBN 978-92-4-150198-9). World Health Organization. Medical device donations: considerations for solicitation and provision. 2011, WHO (ISBN 978-92-4-150140-8).
129. Infra note 151. See also, Johnston J.C., Zebenigus M., on behalf of Global-Neurology®. Improving healthcare access in resource limited areas as a strategy for promoting healthy lives, reducing poverty, and addressing inequalities and challenges to social inclusion. Fifty seventh session of the United Nations Commission for Social Development. New York, NY. 11-21 Feb 2019. E/CN.5/2019/NGO/33.
130. Lahey T. The ethics of clinical research in low and middle income countries. Handbook of Clin Neurol 2013;118:301–13.
131. See, e.g., Nuffield Council on Bioethics. The ethics of research related to healthcare in developing countries. London, UK: Nuffield Council on Bioethics; 2002. World Medical Association. Declaration of Helsinki, ethical principles for medical research involving human subjects. Principle 19. Council for International Organizations of Medical Sciences. CIOMS international ethical guidelines for biomedical research involving human subjects. Geneva 2002.
132. Available at: http://www.efda.gov.et/publication/gcp-guideline/. (Accessed January 8, 2023).
133. Siddiqi OK, Koralnik IJ, Atadzhanov M, et al. Emerging subspecialties in neurology: global health. Neurology 2013;80:e78–80.
134. Available at: www.aan.com/membership/join-an-aan-section-or-community. (Accessed January 6, 2023).
135. Available at: www.wfneurology.org. The other members being the African Academy of Neurology (AFAN), Asian Oceanian Association of Neurology (AOAN), European Academy of Neurology (EAN), Pan American Federation of Neurological Societies (PAFNS), and Pan Arab Union of Neurological Societies (PAUNS). (Accessed January 6, 2023).
136. Available at: https://www.who.int/health-topics/health-equity#tab=tab_1. Provides an overview of health equity including country profiles and various data compilations including a Health Equity Assessment software program. (Accessed January 18, 2023).
137. World Health Organization, Health inequities and their causes. Available at: (www.WHO.int). Accessed January 6, 2023.
138. Supra notes 98, 129.
139. See, generally The global burden of disease study. Lancet 2020;396(10258):1129–306.
140. See also Murray CJL. The global burden of disease study at 30 years. Nat Med 2022;28:2019–26.
141. World Health Organization. Neurological disorders: public health challenges. 2006. (ISBN 9789241563369).
142. Resolution A/RES/70/1. Transforming our world: the 2030 agenda for sustainable development. In: 70th UN General Assembly. United Nations: New York, 2015.
143. Id. at Agenda, SDG 3.8.
144. Supra note 142, Agenda, at SDG 3.4.
145. WHO launches its Global Action Plan for brain health. Lancet Neurol 2022;21(8):671.

146. Supra note 142, Agenda, Declaration, Introduction, Para 4.
147. Available at: https://www.un.org/development/desa/dpad/least-developed-country-category.html. (33 of the 46 least developed nations are in Africa).
148. WHO. *The state of the health work force in the WHO African region.* Geneva, Switzerland: WHO Regional Office for Africa, ISBN 978-929023455-5; 2021.
149. Supra note 142, Agenda, Para 22, 23, and Para 56; SDG 3(d).
150. WHO Fact Sheet No. 323, 2015.
151. Johnston JC. The second summary report on the Addis Ababa University Department of Neurology Residency Training Program. 15 October 2009. World Health Organization, UN ECOSOC on behalf of GlobalNeurology®.
152. Supra note 98.
153. Tafessa A, Johnston JC. From the front lines of Ethiopia: a plea for the global health section to reconsider priorities. Neurol Today 2014;14(16):4.
154. Johnston JC, Zebenigus M, Zenebe G. Global health: advancing North-South partnerships. Med Law 2017;36(2):157.
155. Johnston JC, Zebenigus M, Arda B. Improving healthcare access in sub-Saharan Africa. Med Law 2018;37(2):74–5.
156. Berkowitz AL. Global perspectives. Neurology mission(s) impossible. Neurology 2014;83:1450–1.
157. Siddiqi OK, Brown M, Cooper C, et al. Developing a successful global neurology program. Ann Neurol 2017;81(2):167–70.
158. Johnston JC, Zebenigus M, on behalf of GlobalNeurology®. Advancing health-care access to ensure inclusiveness and equality. New York: United Nations High Level Segment; 2019. E/2019/NGO/70. (Advancing sustainable access to healthcare is a goal broadly reaffirmed by SDG 3, specifically targeted by SDG 3.8, and unconditionally endorsed in SDG 1.3 and the Agenda's Vision 7).
159. Supra note 142, Agenda, SDG 3(c).
160. World Health Organization. Constitution, Article II(o).
161. Supra note 145.
162. Supra notes 98, 129, 158.
163. Bennett S, Glandon D, Rasanathan K. Governing multisectoral action for health in low income and middle income countries: unpacking the problem and rising to the challenge. BMJ Glob Health 2018;3:e000880.
164. The Partners are Berna Arda (Turkey), Roy Beran (Australia), James C. Johnston (New Zealand and USA), Knut Wester (Norway), and Mehila Zebenigus (Ethiopia), with associates in Africa, Asia, Canada, Europe, UK, and US. Thomas P. Sartwelle (USA) serves as legal counsel. (Neurosurgeon Knut Wester is not a co-author because this article is limited to advancing neurology in LMICs which differs significantly from neurosurgery).
165. There are also 8 pediatric neurologists who completed the child neurology portion of training in Italy, Kenya, and South Africa.
166. Atlas: country resources for neurological disorders. 2nd ed. Geneva: WHO; 2017. ISBN 978-92-4-156550-9.
167. See, generally, United Nations Office for South-South Cooperation. See also, Report of Secretary General on State of South-South Cooperation. Available at: (https://unsouthsouth.org/wp-content/uploads/2022/09/SG-Report-on-SSG-2022.pdf).
168. Wilmshurst JM, Morrow B, du Preez A, et al. The African pediatric fellowship program: training in Africa for Africans. Pediatrics 2016;137(1):e20152741. Available at: https://theapfp.org/about.

169. Personal communication, Professor Jo Wilmshurst. (Over 170 health practitioners have been trained with a 95% retention rate in the pediatric disciplines; 13 are child neurologists).

170. Kruk ME, Gage AD, Arsenault C, et al. High-quality health systems in the Sustainable Development Goals era: time for a revolution. The Lancet Global Health Commission 2018;6:e1196–252.

171. Kruk ME, Pate M. The Lancet Global Health Commission on High Quality Health Systems 1 year on: progress on a global imperative. Lancet Global Health 2020; 8(1):E30–2.

172. Lewis T, Kruk ME. The Lancet Global Health Commission on High Quality Health Systems: countries are seizing the quality agenda. J Glob Health Sci 2019; 1(2):e43.

173. Delivering quality health services: a global imperative for universal health coverage. WHO, OECD, International Bank for Reconstruction and Development/The World Bank. ISBN 978-92-4-151390-6 WHO 2018 Available at: https://apps.who.int/iris/bitstream/handle/10665/272465/9789241513906-eng. pdf?ua=1. (Accessed January 22, 2023).

174. Salasky V, Saylor D. Impact of global health electives on neurology trainees. Ann Neurol 2021;89:851–5.

175. Available at: https://blogs.neurology.org/global/continued-development-of-the-american-academy-of-neurology-global-health-section/. (Accessed January 25, 2023).

176. Yarmoshuk AN, Cole DC, Mwangu M, et al. Reciprocity in international interuniversity global health partnerships. High Educ 2020;79:395–414.

177. Umoren RA, James JE, Litzelman DK. Evidence of reciprocity in reports on international partnerships. Edu Res Int 2012;2012:1–7.

178. See, generally, as a resource guide: Consortium of Universities for Global Health (CUGH), CUGH Global Health Education Competencies Tool Kit. 2nd edition. Washington, DC: Consortium of Universities for Global Health (CUGH) Competency Sub-Committee; 2018.

Moving?

Make sure your subscription moves with you!

To notify us of your new address, find your **Clinics Account Number** (located on your mailing label above your name), and contact customer service at:

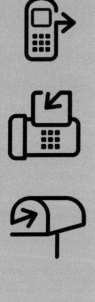

Email: journalscustomerservice-usa@elsevier.com

800-654-2452 (subscribers in the U.S. & Canada)
314-447-8871 (subscribers outside of the U.S. & Canada)

Fax number: 314-447-8029

Elsevier Health Sciences Division
Subscription Customer Service
3251 Riverport Lane
Maryland Heights, MO 63043

*To ensure uninterrupted delivery of your subscription, please notify us at least 4 weeks in advance of move.

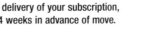

Printed and bound by CPI Group (UK) Ltd, Croydon, CR0 4YY

15/10/2024

01774271-0001